VICTORY OVER DIABETES

Other Keats titles of relevant interest

VICTORY
OVER
DIABETES

A BIO-ECOLOGIC TRIUMPH

William H. Philpott, M.D.
and Dwight K. Kalita, Ph.D.
Introduction by W. D. Currier, M.D.

Keats Publishing, Inc.   New Canaan, Connecticut

Library of Congress Cataloging in Publication Data

Philpott, William H.
    Victory over diabetes.

    Bibliography: p. 262–266
    Includes index.
    1. Diabetes—Nutritional aspects. 2. Orthomolecular therapy.
I. Kalita, Dwight K. II. Title [DNLM: 1. Diabetes mellitus—Drug
therapy. 2. Diabetic diet. 3. Diabetes mellitus—Complications.
4. Cardiovascular diseases—Complications. WK 818 P571v]
RC660.P47 1983   616.4′620654   82-82320
ISBN 0-87983-318-1
ISBN 0-87983-548-6 (pbk.)

Keats Publishing, Inc.
27 Pine Street, New Canaan, Connecticut 06840

Dedication

To those chemical and clinical diabetics who wish to understand the multiple causes of, and through this, the reversal of the degenerative disease process.

Read this first

Bio-Ecologic Medicine is not proposed as a cure-all for diabetes mellitus. Rather, it is advanced as a lifestyle which, when faithfully followed, has the potential of not only reversing a patient's disordered metabolism but also reducing the death-dealing symptoms so associated with the ravages of the diabetes mellitus disease process. This book is designed as a guide to patients undergoing professionally supervised Bio-Ecologic diagnosis and treatment. The information also lends itself to self-help. For obvious reasons, its authors cannot take the medical or legal responsibility of having the contents herein considered as a prescription for anyone. Either you, or the physician who examines and treats you, must take the responsibility for the uses made of this book.

CONTENTS

Acknowledgements

Arthur Coca, M.D., for his observation of maladaptive nonimmunologic foods reversing the disordered carbohydrate metabolism in some diabetics.

Hans Selye, M.D., for outlining the General Adaptation Syndrome which has served well in understanding the basis of the central degenerative disease process in general and diabetes mellitus in particular.

Theron G. Randolph, M.D., for recognizing the reality of food addiction.

John Ely, Ph.D., for observing the role of dehydroascorbic acid in the degenerative disease process in general, and diabetes mellitus in particular.

John Potts, M.D., for providing the statistics which substantiated our clinical observations.

Jon Pangborn, Ph.D., for providing the biochemical understandings of the metabolic disorders of vitamins, minerals, amino acids and essential fatty acids in specific clinical cases of degenerative diseases in general, and diabetes mellitus in particular.

David Horrobin, M.D., for his contribution to the biochemistry of the role of disordered essential fatty acid metabolism in degenerative diseases in general, and in diabetes mellitus in particular.

Thomas Stone, M.D., for confirmation of the chemical and clinical stages of the diabetes mellitus disease process in degenerative disease both physical and mental.

William H. Philpott

I wish to offer an expression of grateful appreciation to my associates at the Bio-Ecologic Research Center Inc., 312 Carpenter Road, Defiance, Ohio 43512, a non-profit, independent, all volunteer organization. Because of the untiring interest and efforts in the production of this book, they have striven far beyond the line of duty in the research and every other step of the process necessary to produce the final draft. I would also like to offer grateful appreciation to Steve Blechman, research scientist, for his contributions to Chapter 11, "EPA, GLA and Prostaglandins."

Dwight K. Kalita

INTRODUCTION

This book opens new and fundamental vistas for physician and layman alike. It describes accurately and succinctly important, not yet realized errors of chemistry and lifestyle that are responsible for perversions of glucose metabolism, ranging from hypoglycemia to hyperglycemia. Today, insulin injections and a low refined carbohydrate, low fat diet for the treatment of diabetes is so inadequate that it almost borders on malpractice. The authors have detailed holistic diagnostic procedures and have offered indispensable modes of treatment that most physicians would not conceive as being necessary and important. Those who read this book will become informed concerning the staggering amount of biochemical individuality in all of us.

Who should read this book? To me the number one reader should be the medical students while their minds are still open and flexible. The next most important reader perhaps should be the layman. He will not only learn what diagnostic and treatment procedures he should expect from his practicing physician, but by becoming broadly and highly informed, he will not let the rigid, unknowing physician intimidate him.

The doctors who have written this book outline mental and physical infirmities that result from blood sugar inequities. Blood sugar is the fuel of all body chemistry. Our brain requires 30 percent more glucose and oxygen than other parts of the body. If the brain becomes starved for blood sugar, or if there is inadequate insulin to carry the glucose into every one of the sixty or more trillion cells of our body, a large variety of illnesses can result, particularly those that involve the brain. Drs. Philpott and Kalita also cover Bio-Ecologic treatment methods of reversing these infirmities.

One of the most common complaints of my patients is that, "All my doctor does is prescribe drugs, and he gets angry if I ask questions, especially questions about diet and vitamins." All too often the physician says in essence, "I don't believe in vitamins. Just get your nutrition from the good old American diet." In such cases he certainly has a great deal more confidence in the American diet than I do. This book, among so many other things, is an instruction course concerning proper nutrition and supplements indicated for the diabetic and hypoglycemic patient. An educated patient is always a more successfully treated patient. It is the responsibility of the physician to find the causes and recommend corrections for the errors of living which produce essentially all disease. We all partake of these errors, each in our own ways. They include: smoking, drinking, drugs, coffee, tea, insufficient exercise, sleep or rest, emotional and/or environmental stresses and tensions, traumatic injuries such as accidents or surgery, nutritional deficiencies, errors of eating, and so on.

Drs. Philpott and Kalita stress the fundamental truth that the patient must cure himself with the doctor's assistance. It's the "doctor within" the patients that must get them well and keep them well. The "doctor within" knows much more how to "cure" a patient than the doctor knows, but the patient must be sure that he supplies to the "doctor within" all the necessary instruments and tools to work within the form of ideal nutrition and ideal body chemistry. He must also be sure he doesn't intoxicate or nutritionally starve the "doctor within." It is pleasing and gratifying to the patient to learn that he can, to a very high degree, take charge of his own processes of getting well. For those physicians who practice nutritional, metabolic, preventive, holistic, orthomolecular or Bio-Ecologic medicine, great personal satisfaction often arises out of their practice of medicine because most of their patients do indeed get well!

W.D. Currier, M.D.

A Breakthrough in Magnetic Energy Healing

Central to non-insulin dependent diabetes (Type II diabetes) is insulin resistance. Over the past 20 years I have tested several thousand patients for disordered carbohydrate metabolism in relationship to single food test meals. Several hundred of these were also tested for insulin response to single food test meals which were correlated with the degree of carbohydrate disorder. The primary diagnoses of these patients were a wide spectrum of physical and mental disorders including several hundred maturity-onset diabetics and a few insulin-dependent juvenile diabetics. From these studies solid evidence emerged that the insulin resistance of Type II non-insulin dependent diabetes mellitus is produced by maladaptive reactions largely to foods and, to a lesser extent, to common environmental chemicals such as car exhaust. These maladaptive reactions consisted of an assortment of IgG food allergies, food addictions, ill-defined food intolerances, hypersensitivity and toxic reactions to environmental chemicals.

There is a routine clearance of insulin resistance as well

as the carbohydrate disorder with avoidance of the foods and substances evoking the maladaptive reactions. The reactions consist of an array of physical and emotional symptoms, as well as higher-than-normal blood sugar response. The carbohydrate disorder of brief duration and the chronic carbohydrate disorders justifying the diagnosis of diabetes mellitus Type II behave alike and therefore it is concluded that Type II diabetes is simply an extension of these lesser carbohydrate disorders. Both are readily reversed by avoidance of the maladaptive reactive substances, followed by carefully spaced exposure to them.

Unfortunately, there is a low level of awareness of the ecologic causes of insulin-resistant carbohydrate disorder. The stress of obesity has been highlighted since some 80 percent of diabetics at the time of their onset are obese. This obesity certainly is a significant stress that should be corrected. However, and surprisingly, the insulin resistance and the carbohydrate disorder were corrected *immediately* by avoidance and spacing *before* there was any time for weight reduction to have occurred. It is strange that in scientific medicine this is so little known, especially since a statistical verification has been published in the right place, that is, the journal *Diabetes*.

For years the presence and level of hormones and enzymes have been believed to be the producers of biological reactions without any consideration of an energy source which could make such reactions possible. This belief in spontaneously occurring biological responses is no longer tenable now that we understand the role of electromagnetics. Specifically, magnetism creates the energy which makes biological response possible.

For years it was customary to consider magnetism as one unit of energy. However, it has been conclusively demonstrated that magnetism is two energies that have opposite biological effects when these energies are separated. The balance between these two energies governs metabolism. Magnetism is a push and pull system. The clockwise spin of a positive magnetic field pushes while the counter-clockwise spin of the negative magnetic field pulls.

Negative magnetic fields and positive magnetic fields are both magnetic energy, with 180-degrees opposite response in biological systems. Life energy is the balance between these two systems. An example is acid-base balance. The positive magnetic pole is acidifying and the negative magnetic pole is alkalizing in terms of biological response to single magnetic fields from a unipoled magnet. Biological life has a balance between acidity and alkalinity.

Another important issue is the demonstrated evidence that the positive magnetic pole evokes inflammation and the negative magnetic pole is anti-inflammatory and inflammatory resolving. Understanding the oppositeness of biological responses evoked by the separate magnetic fields is critically important. Exposing tissues to single magnetic poles can produce a predictable biological response in those tissues. I routinely correlate saliva pH with maladaptive reactions to foods and chemicals. These reactions are routinely acid and can be controlled by a negative magnetic field. Inflammation is characteristically an aspect of degenerative diseases and can be controlled by exposure to a negative magnetic field.

How is insulin resistance caused by maladaptive reactions to foods, chemicals and inhalants? The formulation is on this order: These maladaptive reactions—whether allergic, addictive, toxic or otherwise unexplainable inflammatory reactions—cause an inflammatory edema of cells and whole tissue groups. Insulin's assignment is to carry blood glucose through the cell wall into the cell. A cell with a swollen membrane cannot make proper use of insulin; thus the blood sugar remains in the blood and is not transferred into the cell. When these cells or tissues are placed in a negative magnetic field, the inflammatory edema is corrected and insulin works as it should. Therefore, not only should we use avoidance and spacing of maladaptive-reacting substances, but also tissue exposure to negative magnetic field energy to correct the insulin resistance of maturity-onset diabetes mellitus. Exposure to negative magnetic field energy ahead of a meal has been conclusively demonstrated effective in reducing the chances of a

---

maladaptive reaction to foods. Maladaptive reactions to most environmental substances are essentially the same process as maladaptive reactions to foods.

The inflammatory reactions which occur due to the diabetes mellitus disease process reduce oxygen to tissues, encourage invasion of microorganisms (viruses, fungi and bacteria), produce inflammation of arteries with atheromatus build-up and many other tissue and nerve degenerative disorders. Great advances have been made in scientific medicine in understanding these degenerative disease processes. However, the most important thing we understand today is that this process exists because there is an imbalance between the positive and negative magnetic poles where positive magnetic energy has the ascendancy over the negative magnetic energy. Direct tissue exposure to negative magnetic energy can do much to correct this magnetic energy imbalance disorder.

—William H. Philpott, M.D.

VICTORY OVER DIABETES

CHAPTER ONE

Diabetes: The need for a nutritional approach

The following is a statement delivered by Mr. Thomas J. Watson, Jr., chairman of the Executive Committee of the International Business Machine Corporation (IBM) at the Mayo Clinic in Rochester, Minnesota, on November 19, 1970.

Let me start by asking a question that this great medical center brings to mind: How would you like to live in a country which, according to the figures available in the United States during the past two decades:

> *has dropped from seventh in the world to sixteenth in the prevention of infant mortality; has dropped in female life expectancy from sixth to eighth; has dropped in male life expectancy from tenth to twenty-fourth; and which has brought itself this unenviable trend by spending more of its gross national product for medical care ($1.00 out of every $14.00) than any other country on the face of the earth?*

You know the country I am talking about: our own U.S.A., the home of the free, the home of the brave, and the home of a decrepit, inefficient, high-priced system of medical care. Just

*look for a moment at what some of the figures mean. They mean
that in infant mortality we have been overtaken by France, the
U.K. and Japan, that in male life expectancy we have been
overtaken by France, Japan, West Germany and Italy. I know
experts can disagree over precise international standing. And I
realize that medical problems in the United States, Europe and
Japan are not identical. But the evidence overwhelmingly indicates
that we are falling down on the job, heading in the wrong
direction, and becoming as a nation a massive medical disgrace.*[1]

The plethora of these figures given to us by the
chairman of IBM reveals the sad fact that the business of
health care in our nation is the fastest growing failing
business in these United States. In fact, a close examination
of the figures on the incidence of degenerative disease in
our nation discloses the deplorable situation that really
exists. Two of the major degenerative diseases, for example,
that are destroying the lives of countless numbers of
Americans every year are diabetes and heart disease.
Between 1965 and 1973, the prevalence of diabetes increased
more than 50 percent in the United States, according
to the National Commission on Diabetes established by the
United States Congress in 1974. In 1974 alone, more than
600,000 new cases of diabetes and its complications were
responsible for more than 300,000 deaths annually, making
it the third ranking category on the list of killer
diseases. Diabetes, in short, is a major health problem in
the United States. It directly affects 10 million Americans,
and anyone born today who lives an average life span of
seventy years has greater than a one in five chance of
developing this killer disease! The economic toll of diabetes
alone, without even considering its complications, is estimated
to be $5.4 billion every year.

More disheartening facts about diabetes indicate that
women are 50 percent more likely than men to have the
disease; nonwhites are one fifth more likely than whites to
have it, and poor people (incomes less than $5,000 per
year) are three times as likely as middle income and
wealthy individuals to have the disorder. During pregnancy,

diabetes increases the chances of premature delivery and even death of the baby. It is the third major chronic disease among children as well as the most common endocrine disorder among young people. Diabetics are twenty-five times more prone to gangrene—often leading to amputation—and six times as prone to heart disease. Tragically, the life expectancy of a diabetic is approximately one third less than that of the general population.

Heart disease, statistically speaking, is very closely related to the incidence of diabetes. While diabetes ranks third in our nation as the cause of death, heart disease is the largest killer and accounts for 53 percent of all deaths. A staggering 726,000 people died of heart disease in 1976, with cancer ranking a distant second, claiming about half that many lives. Today, in the 1980s, arteriosclerosis is the most common form of heart disease, and claims over 900,000 lives each year in the U.S.A.

But the connection between diabetes and arteriosclerosis (heart disease) is not only a statistical one. As we shall see, so close, metabolically speaking, is the association between diabetes and the cardiovascular and cerebrovascular complications of arteriosclerosis, that a number of physicians and scientists are beginning to ask whether these complications that eventually deteriorate into a full-blown heart attack and/or stroke are not in fact actually part of the diabetic disease process. Much more explanation of the diabetic disease process and its connection with heart disease will, of course, be forthcoming, but for now, let us keep in mind the idea that all too often insulin-requiring "controlled" diabetics develop a thickening of the tiny blood vessels (capillaries) which nourish numerous tissues of the body. Those blood vessels most seriously affected by the disease process are the capillaries of the kidneys and eyes. Blood vessel disease in diabetics can also, however, lead to gangrene in the legs and feet. But worst of all, when the coronary circulation system of the heart is involved, its life-giving blood vessels may eventually close up with deposits of death-dealing metabolic debris. The end result is a heart attack; if the blood vessels that supply the brain are involved, a stroke usually ensues.

When insulin was discovered in 1922, diabetes was considered to be merely a deficiency of this chemical substance. Accordingly, since insulin was now available, diabetes was thought to be a cured disease by most doctors. The thinking then was—and these ideas unfortunately still persist in the modern medical world of today—that if an individual diabetic was deficient in the pancreatic hormone named insulin, a substance which is needed for the normal metabolism of blood sugar in the body, the consequence of this was that the patient's body did not make proper use of the sugar and starches that were ingested; blood sugar thus accumulated in the body in levels that were unacceptable and ultimately spilled over into the urine. Most medical people at the time were certain in their belief that this condition was effectively treated by the single, often daily, administration of insulin injections which would in turn make up for any deficiency. The cause of this deficiency and why it developed in the first place was, at the time, not medically agreed upon. In fact, an answer to the question was not all that important since the symptomatic relief of an insulin deficiency was a simple matter of daily injections of the hormone.

However, as the years progressed, physicians began discovering that while they were indeed controlling body sugar levels by the use of insulin injections, other associated complications began introducing themselves with disturbing regularity. It slowly became apparent, based on the horrendous complications developed by insulin-requiring diabetics—involving the eyes and kidneys, the peripheral nerves and tiny blood vessels all over the body, the coronary circulation system, the brain and so forth—that something was, and still is, radically wrong with the conventional approach to treating the disease.

Back in the 1890s people with diabetes died most of the time (63.8 percent) because their sugar levels were not being controlled; hence, they experienced death-dealing comas. However, this pattern of death was dramatically altered with the introduction of insulin in 1922. Coma deaths dropped from 63.8 percent to 41.5 percent by 1922 and then even more so (to 8.3 percent) by 1936. In 1968, only 1 percent of diabetics died from coma. However, as one statistical curve was descending, another curve was ascending, namely diabetic deaths due to cardiorenal-vascular, arteriosclerotic complications. In 1897 only 17.5 percent died from this cause; but by 1968 the figures skyrocketed to a staggering 74.2 percent.

What all this means for today's insulin-requiring "controlled" diabetic is that he or she will probably live just a long enough life to develop greater susceptibility either to infectious diseases, kidney problems, cardiovascular complications which can deteriorate into retinopathy, arteriosclerosis or a heart attack, and/or to cerebrovascular complications which can cause a stroke. This obviously is not a very encouraging picture! Gloomy indeed it is, but at least a growing number of concerned physicians are becoming increasingly aware of the fact that new and more effective approaches to the treatment of diabetes are very urgently needed. "The name of the game in diabetic research," writes Bernard E. Lowenstein, M.D., "must become the prevention of the vascular and neurological complications of diabetes. A growing portion of the medical profession now realizes that neither insulin nor oral anti-diabetic agents, nor diets as now used, can do this job. Diabetes remains an unbridled killer and maimer, and the notion that it is controllable remains a myth."[2]

Related to these previously mentioned ideas, the results of a study of life expectancies among physicians reported by the American Medical Association further suggest the urgency in developing more effective diabetic treatment methodologies. Among doctors, the death rate from diabetes was reported to be 35 percent higher than that of the laymen. "If doctors die from diabetes more often than do laymen," reasons Dr. Lowenstein, "maybe it is because the accepted methods of treating diabetes are at fault. Since doctors are more likely to follow these methods religiously, maybe that is why they are more apt to die from them than laymen are!"[3] This quotation is a very strong indictment of physicians who still practice the conventional approach to diabetes. Let it be added, however, that we hope the reader, after reviewing the full contents of this book, will see the validity of this indictment.

Let us concede, then, that the truly significant problem with which the physician is confronted in helping the diabetic is the fact that the patient is literally "sick all over." No longer, therefore, can treatment be restricted to reducing the levels of sugar in the blood or improving only the metabolism of glucose (blood sugar) in various tissues of the body. This does not mean, however, that the degradation of glucose metabolism is not still a major issue; it is indeed the one problem which requires our immediate and most serious attention. For unless the metabolism of glucose is supported in the right way, there can be no remedy for diabetic trends or development. But the answer to the total diabetic dilemma lies in following a comprehensive, constructive program which supports all the normal body activities; such a program must be designed to eliminate improper metabolism as well as *all* the associated complications accompanying the diabetic disease process.

To begin to appreciate the staggering complexity of the problem we are discussing, we should start by understanding the biochemical complexity of the human body—an organism which is regulated by uncountable balancing forces in every one of its trillions of cells. Considering that there are reported to be, for example, more than five thousand enzyme reactions in each of our trillions of cells every microsecond of our lives, and that each enzyme controls the synthesis or degradation of at least one chemical process in the body, any single concept that we might try to grasp of the wondrous biochemical world within each of us would really be hopeless and beyond our wildest imaginations. What we can and must do here at the onset is appreciate, in a very general fashion, Nature's complex plan for proper sugar metabolism.

Upon examining the subsequent chapters, it is hoped

the reader will develop: 1. a general appreciation of precisely how complicated our biochemical being is; 2. a knowledge of what pathways nature has provided for the utilization of glucose in the human body; 3. an awareness that whatever interferes with these operations leads to degenerative disease; 4. an understanding that there are no so-called drugs anywhere in these biochemical processes; and 5. a conviction that the necessary ingredients for all these processes of metabolizing glucose are only substances or chemicals which nature has established and which are needed for proper functioning. These substances are: vitamins, minerals, trace elements, amino acids, essential fatty acids, hormones and enzymes! The assumption being presented here is that if all these substances involved in the correct metabolism of glucose are present in the concentrations nature has intended, there will be no diabetic problem. Hence, the most effective prevention and treatment of diabetes and its associated complication of symptoms involves the consistent and professional management of all the necessary vitamins, minerals, trace elements, amino acids, essential fatty acids, hormones and enzymes which nature requires.

Thus, what we need to do is study the interactions and balancing mechanisms existing among these substances or chemicals much more completely and carefully than before, so that we may more accurately gauge the degree and types of damage inflicted by man upon nature's biochemical pathways to optimum health and resistance to disease. Obviously, this task must involve an in-depth study and complete examination of the field of nutrition and its relationship to degenerative diseases. So far, modern medicine has failed to accomplish this urgent task.

Senator George McGovern asked the question of Dr. Philip R. Lee, director of the health policy program at the School of Medicine, University of California at San Francisco: "Are the graduates that are coming out of our medical schools now, that is, the doctors that are going to go out and practice and deal with patients, are they properly trained in your judgment on the importance of nutrition in overall human development?" Dr. Lee replied: "Absolutely

not. They know more about heart transplants than they do
about basic nutrition. The technology that has so taken hold
of medicine has sort of obsessed us all, and we instruct
students in all kinds of technological advances. But in very
basic things, like what is an adequate diet, we do not do
an adequate job. In the medical schools of the country, we
are devoting tremendous resources to pediatric prenatal
intensive care units to care for infants of mothers who are
given inadequate nutrition counseling during their pregnancy. That is largely the fault of our own neglect of
nutrition counseling in health care. I would guess 90
percent of the graduates of our medical schools couldn't
describe an adequate nutritious diet that was appropriate
for people at various stages of life."[4] On the basis of the
statement made by Dr. Lee, and those by other physicians
as well, a high percentage of lay people have developed a
mood of disquietude after learning how few doctors are
aware of the advantages of nutrient therapy in the treatment
of degenerative disease. "The Oriental physicians of
antiquity," writes Dr. B.E. Lowenstein, "probably knew
far more about foods and what they do to the body than
the twentieth century U.S. doctor with all the benefits of
modern scientific knowledge. Even worse, the typical
doctor in private practice or hospital practice today doesn't
even care very much about nutrition. It is much easier to
prescribe drugs in a hurry than to sit down and figure out
just what the right therapeutic diet would be for each
individual patient and his particular problem."[5]

Two thousand five hundred years ago, Hippocrates,
the Father of Medicine, said to his medical students: "Let
thy food be thy medicine and thy medicine be thy food."
Moses Maimonides, the great twelfth century physician of
the sultan, repeated the Hippocratic sentiment when he
said: "No illness which can be treated by diet should be
treated by any other means." In essence, what Hippocrates
and Maimonides were insisting was that their medical
students practice nutrient therapy. This particular type of
medical therapy is being practiced by physicians today,
even though only a minority of doctors is using it. It is

reported, however, that there is a rapidly developing rebirth of interest in this unique type of medical orientation, and physicians from all around the world are beginning to look more closely at the wisdom of the Father of Medicine.

Today, nutrient therapy is basically composed of two medical disciplines: Orthomolecular Medicine and Human Ecology. The term "Orthomolecular Medicine" was first coined in 1968 by Linus Pauling, Ph.D., twice Nobel Prize winner. The word means "right molecule." A deeper understanding of the meaning of the word has some very interesting implications. First of all, Orthomolecular physicians believe that the treatment of infectious and degenerative diseases should be a matter of varying the concentration of substances or "right molecules": (i.e., vitamins, minerals, trace elements, amino acids, enzymes, essential fatty acids, hormones, including insulin, and so on) which are normally present in the human body. This notion implies that the nutritional micro-environment of every single cell in our body is extremely important to our optimum health, and that deficiencies in this environment constitute the major cause of disease. If deficiencies in the cell develop, then the thinking is that the concentration of these chemicals needed for optimum health must be altered in accordance with the individual needs. The assumption here is that if the biochemical individual integrity of each and every cell of our bodies is nourished with the optimum nutrients, enzymes or hormones necessary for their proper and healthy functioning, then the internal environment can be brought into line with individual human needs, and chronic degenerative diseases will eventually be controlled.

Obviously, the list of these necessary right molecules is the same for every human being, but the relative amounts needed by each individual are as distinctively different as fingerprints. Why? you ask. Because the kind of diet you eat, the relative amounts of physical, mental, and emotional stress you have, the particular environment in which you live and work, the unique individually determined biochemical heredity pattern you are given, the type of soil in which your food is grown, the type of water you drink,

the amount of exercise you have, all add up to determine
the fact that your body is not a bunch of cells needing a
"one for all and all for one" minimum daily requirement.
You are a distinctively unique individual with unique
biochemical needs. If your body cells are ailing, as they
certainly must be in any form of human disease, then
chances are good that it is because they are not being
adequately provisioned with the optimum nutrients,
enzymes or hormones they need to sustain and propagate
healthy human tissues, organs and life in general. In other
words, cellular health is not based on a minimum daily
requirement but on an optimum daily need, individually
determined by your own biochemical uniqueness. And this
is precisely where Orthomolecular Medicine comes to the
front lines in the battle against disease. Many medical men
are beginning to observe clinically positive results when
their patients are treated at the cellular level with biological
weapons that nature has provided in her own structure of
defense since the beginning of time.

The other equally important side of Nutrient Therapy
is called Human Ecology. Human ecologists scientifically
examine man's environment in order to discover sources
of environmentally produced illness. The word "environment"
is here used in a very broad sense. It includes every
chemical and food with which a person may come in
contact. This notion means that the field of allergy is
much larger than the traditional immunologists have projected
for it. There are many maladaptive, allergic-like reactions,
including radical shifts in normal blood sugar levels as
well as central nervous system reactions, that do not
manifest antibody formation and, therefore, do not fit the
immunologist's rather narrow definition of allergy. Clinical
Ecology is a more inclusive term and includes all maladaptive
reactions, physical, mental, emotional or otherwise,
occurring on exposure to any substance, be it a food,
chemical or pollutant. As a group of susceptible patients
were subjected to ecologically oriented testing methods,
evaluations and diagnosis, the following progressive levels
of reactions were recorded: 1. acute localized physical

effects (rhinitis, bronchitis, asthma, eczema and gastro-intestinal and other allergies); 2. acute systemic effects (headache, fatigue, myalgia, arthralgia, neuralgia, hyper-glycemia (diabetes), hypoglycemia and other generalized physical syndromes); 3. acute mental effects (confusion, depression, delusions, hallucinations and other advanced cerebral and behavioral abnormalities). As these chronic symptoms were studied by means of comprehensive environmental control, clinically induced reexposures to the incriminating substances gave predictable results. It was during the course of these clinical experiences that the dominant role of chemical and food allergies in producing "ecologic" physical and mental illnesses became apparent. Now physicians discovered that they were indeed dealing with the etiology or root causes of many of their patients' illnesses.

By contrast, Toximolecular Medicine, a type of therapy used by the majority of physicians in our country for only the past forty years, is the administration of drugs at sublethal levels. Drugs, of course, are alien chemicals which are not normally present in the cellular structure of the human body. They radically alter man's biochemical-physiological internal environment and often trigger very severe side effects which can indeed be dangerous. Needless to say, drugs do not cure or prevent the disease process, especially degenerative disease; rather, they offer—at best—symptomatic relief, while the fundamental underlying disease process continues uninterrupted. "The basic fault of these weapons [drugs]," writes Dr. Roger Williams, "is that they have no known connection with the disease process itself. . . . Drugs are wholly unlike nature's weapons. . . . They tend to mask the difficulty, not eliminate it. They contaminate the internal environment (with side effects), create dependence on the part of the patient, and often complicate the physician's job by erasing valuable clues as to the real source of the trouble."[6]

A good example that illustrates the validity of Dr. Williams's observation is the current medical use of oral diabetic drugs. There are two basic types of oral drugs.

1. Sulfonylureas, which include tolbutamide (Orinase), chlorpropamide (Diabinese), tolayamide (Tolinase). These drugs produce a lowering of the blood glucose by stimulating the release of insulin from the patient's own pancreas. It follows that for the drugs to be effective, the patient's pancreas must itself be able to make enough insulin. 2. The other basic type of oral diabetic drug is biguanides. The chief example of this general drug classification is phenformin (DBI, Metrol). It is still not clear how the biguanide drugs work. Some theories suggest they increase the utilization of blood glucose by muscle and other tissues, and others state that they slow down the rate of absorption of carbohydrates from the bowel. If seen in the light of Dr.Williams's statement concerning drugs, it is more understandable why phenformin was banned in the United States in 1977, following HEW Secretary Califano's order to stop all sales of this harmful synthetic chemical on July 23, 1977. Until it was taken off the market in that year, phenformin was the only member of the biguanide drug family available in this country. Prior to its ban, people were suffering such side effects as nausea, vomiting, diarrhea and loss of appetite. The drug's most dangerous side effect, however, is a disease called lactic acidosis. This is a condition in which lactic acid, formed when cells break down glucose without oxygen, is produced in excess and becomes extremely toxic to the body. The initial symptomatology of this disorder includes vomiting, weakness and nausea, but gradually, if this drug therapy is continued, the patient loses consciousness and can fall into a coma. Death occurs in about half of the lactic acidosis cases,[7] but estimates have ranged as high as 62.5 percent.[8] The Food and Drug Administration, that governmental agency which is supposed to "protect the consumer" from dangerous foods and drugs like phenformin, moved slowly against this particular drug. Despite the FDA's Bureau of Drugs estimate that phenformin-induced lactic acidosis would cause fifty to seven hundred deaths annually,[9] it took a special petition and law suit from the Health Research Group, a consumer advocacy group, to persuade HEW Secretary

Califano to withdraw phenformin from the market as an imminent health hazard.

But what about the other oral diabetic drugs, sulfonylureas, used in our country today? Are they truly effective and safe for the consumer? According to S.M. Wolfe, M.D., and a large-scale University Group Diabetes Program (UGDP), the answer to these questions is an emphatic "NO!" Writes Dr. Wolfe, "Since 1969, the medical community has had evidence that these drugs (tolbutamide, chlorpropamide and tolayamide) double the yearly death rate by heart and blood vessel disease in maturity-onset diabetics who use them. At that time the University Group Diabetes Program (UGDP) released results of a large-scale study commissioned by the National Institute of Health and carried out by diabetes experts at twelve clinics in the U.S. and Puerto Rico. After eight years of research, the results showed that oral hypoglycemic agents caused one excess cardiovascular death per 100 maturity-onset diabetics taking the medication per year. Over a period of ten years this meant that the oral hypoglycemic agents doubled the death rate from cardiovascular causes. This translates into the fact that these drugs could be causing 10,000 to 15,000 unnecessary deaths in this country alone every year."[10] If the use of any drug in the treatment of diabetes is to be considered an effective treatment modality, it should, without any question of doubt, not only lower blood glucose levels in the patient and do so in a reliable fashion, but it should also prevent or delay the appearance of any associated complications and thus prolong health and life in general. Since, according to the overwhelming scientific evidence of recent studies,[11] both sulfonylureas and biguanides actually shorten life expectancy, create a greater degree of serious side-effect complications, and do not lower the blood glucose levels in an optimal fashion for the majority of patients, neither of these general drug classifications should be considered an effective therapy. Therefore, if you are taking an oral diabetic drug ("hypoglycemic agent"), chances are good it may be harmful to you; the chances are even better that it can't help you. This statement is especially true in light of some of the more effective nontoxic treatment modalities used by Orthomolecular-Ecologic physicians.

It should not surprise anyone to learn that even toximolecular physicians are beginning to see the truth concerning the mounting negative evidence of oral diabetic drugs. According to Dr. Wolfe,

After a peak in 1973, however, the use of oral agents has shown an encouraging rapid descent. The most recent data from 1977 show a decrease of about ten million prescriptions a year from 1973 or a fall of more than 50 percent, even though hundreds of thousands of new cases of diabetes are diagnosed each year by screening programs. What this means is that approximately 1,741,000 patients formerly taking hypoglycemics have switched to a safer therapy, but 1-¾ million haven't. . . .

This dramatic decline shows that doctors are beginning to believe the studies which have proven oral hypoglycemic drugs unsafe and ineffective in the long run and that some of the medical profession is rediscovering safer treatments for diabetes. However, the fact that over nine and a half million prescriptions were written for oral hypoglycemic drugs in 1977 demonstrates that the oral agents nevertheless remain in widespread use. Oral hypoglycemic drugs still command giant-sized profits for their manufacturers. Since the drugs appeared twenty years ago, U.S. consumers have paid more than $2 billion for them. That phenformin stayed on the market as long as it did, despite scientific evidence against it, and that other oral agents have remained high volume drugs are due to three main reasons— doctors' pride, drug companies' profits, and the reluctance of the Food and Drug Administration to take steps against the oral agents.[12]

Indeed, in financial terms, the United States spends over $200 million annually for oral hypoglycemic drugs. Obviously, the drug companies that make large profits on the overuse of these fundamentally unsafe and, in the long run, ineffective drugs have an important stake in protecting their profits. They use indirect but powerful tactics to accomplish these ends. For example, drug companies are on record for spending $5,000 per doctor per year[13] strictly on promotional materials that "educate" the physician on their drugs for sale. In the light of such large expenditures of sales promotion money, it is understandable that many doctors, without even being aware of it, are unduly influenced by these advertising messages. Furthermore, all too often physicians are simply too busy with their work to research in an in-depth fashion all the up to date, independently studied, published clinical experiments on this or that drug; so they are forced to rely, in the main, upon the sales promotion men from the drug companies as their major source of information concerning new and old products on the market. Obviously, since there are vested interests involved here, this type of information may not always be reliable.

But why, you might ask, if antidiabetic drugs are so fundamentally ineffective and unsafe to use, are the majority of physicians in our country still oriented toward the toximolecular approach in medicine in treating this killer disease? Is it strictly because the large drug companies are so persuasive in the sales promotion, or are there other factors involved? An answer comes in part from the hearing before the Select Committee on Nutrition and Human Needs of the United States Senate on June 22, 1977.

Senator George McGovern: *Achieving recognition of the relationship between nutrition and health is still very much a struggle. Established scientific thinking remains weighted against those few scientists and practitioners who are striving to understand the complex links between the food we consume and how we think and behave as individuals.*

Senator McGovern to Dr. Mike Lesser: *With the methods we are now using are we not simply adding to the burden of the hospitals and perpetuating a system of therapy (i.e., Toximolecular) that may help the drug industry but really is not dealing with the basic problem?*

Dr. Lesser: *I believe we are. I believe that is the situation. We are just providing symptomatic relief and control at this moment and not getting at the basic cause. Tranquilizers came out in the fifties. Fortunately, or unfortunately, for the treatment of mental illness, tranquilizers are drugs, and therefore patentable substances. In other words, a pharmaceutical house can receive an exclusive monopoly to produce that particular substance for, I believe, 10 years. This allows the company to make money*

off that drug. This money pays for research into further use
of drugs. It also pays to hire detail men to visit physicians
who are treating patients, and every physician in this country
is currently visited by detail men who tell him about the latest drug
discoveries. . . . It also pays for the testing necessary in order to
receive Federal Government approval to use those drugs. . . .
Vitamins (all nutrients) are not patentable substances. Nutrients
are available in nature and no one can patent them.

Senator Schweiker: The FDA tried to ban them a year and a
half ago. We had to fight that.

Dr. Lesser: The physicians in medical school are taught to use
drugs, not nutrients. Hours are spent teaching physicians how to
prescribe various drugs to treat disease.

Senator Schweiker: How can we change that? I am very
concerned about that!

Dr. Lesser: Clinical nutrition should be a mandatory course in
every medical school. (Applause)

Senator Schweiker: Last time we did a rough check it was
something like 10 medical schools at the most that had a
department of nutrition teaching applied nutrition, and that was
giving the benefit of the doubt. Less than 10 percent even had a
functioning department in the area.

Dr. Lesser: There is a good deal of nutrition used in medicine.
Unfortunately, it is not identified as the front-line treatment, the
way that Hippocrates and Maimonides thought of nutrition.
Within the last 30 or 40 years, with the advent of drugs, drugs
have become the front-line treatment of illness in general. But I
believe that with the development of increased interest in
nutrition and Orthomolecular Medicine, this picture will change.
Nutrient therapy has distinct advantages. It is less expensive as
nutrients are not patentable. They are less expensive than drugs.
Certainly they are safer. They are safer because they are natural
substances which are normally present in the body and are not
foreign to the body, and our bodies have evolved over millions
of years, and they have evolved with nutrients. Nutrients are
absolutely necessary to life. Even when you give them in rather
large quantities, they are generally without any side effects. I
think nutrient therapy is more effective because it is getting at
the cause of the problem.[14]

Nutrient therapy, or as it will be termed in subsequent
chapters, "Bio-Ecologic Medicine" (so named by Marshall

Mandell, M.D.), is more effective than toximolecular therapy because it recognizes that a healthy body is based on healthy cells. And all the cells in our body have the foundation of their very existence in vitamins, minerals, trace elements, amino acids, enzymes, and so forth, the very same nutrients used by Bio-Ecologic physicians. These physicians are interested in a very broad spectrum of biological, nutritional, ecologic and metabolic disorders and the interrelationships existing among these disorders. In short, they are more interested in curing and preventing the causes of disease than in mere symptomatic treatment and relief. If they fail at this task, then the medical field will not be the third largest industry in our country, as it is today, but it will be number one. If this tragedy ever occurs, and statistical analysis suggests it well might do so by the year 2000, then it will take the entire Gross National Product to support its existence—an absurd thought to imagine! Bio-Ecologic Medicine, on the other hand, is a safe, economical, prevention-oriented and, as we shall see, effective alternative to our current medical crisis. "There is no reason," concludes Dr. Bressler, "to use a drug that does not work. Even the safest drug is of no value if it has no efficacy. The long-term effectiveness of controlling blood sugar by oral hypoglycemic agents is minimal. In the studies of both Feldman and the UGDP, there was no noteworthy lowering of blood glucose. . . . Therefore, at present, oral hypoglycemic agents have no demonstrated useful role in the management of maturity-onset diabetes."[15]

REFERENCES

1. *Proceedings of the San Diego Biomedical Symposium.* 1974. 13:31–39.

2. Lowenstein, B. E. 1976. *Diabetes.* New York: Harper and Row, p. 227.

3. ———. *Diabetes*, p. 18.

4. Borrmann, W. R. 1979. *Comprehensive Answers to Nutrition.* Chicago: New Horizons Publishing, p. 5.

5. Lowenstein, B. E. *Diabetes*, p. 68.

6. Williams, R. J. 1971. *Nutrition Against Disease*. New York: Pitman, p. 11.

7. Forbath, N. 1977. *Primary Care* 4(4):629–639.

8. *Scrip*. April 30, 1977, p. 16.

9. *FDA Drug Bulletin*. 1977. 7(3):4.

10. Wolfe, S. M. 1978. *Off Diabetes Pills*. Washington: Public Citizen's Health Research Group, p. 9.

11. Ricketts, H. T. 1970. *Diabetes* 19 (suppl. 2):IV; AMA Council on Drugs. 1970. *Diabetes* 19 (suppl. 2):VII; Edwards, C. C. 1970. *Diabetes* 19 (suppl. 2):VIII; Chalmers, T. C. 1975. *JAMA* 231:624–625; *Federal Register* (July 7, 1975) 40(130):28588; *Diabetes* 19 (suppl. 2): 789–830; UGDP. 1971. *JAMA* 218:1400–1410; UGDP. 1971. *JAMA* 217: 777–784; UGDP. 1976. *Diabetes* 25(12):1129–1151; Hadden, D. R. 1972. *Lancet* 1:335–338; Boyle, D. 1972. *Lancet* 1:338–339; Soler, N. G. 1974. *Lancet* 1:475–477; Haider, H. April 1975. *Clinical Research* 22(3):215A; Reid, N. 1970. *British Medical Bulletin* 26(3):191; Kurihara, T. 1971. *Diabetes Mellitus in Asia*, p. 24; Knussman, D. 1971. *Das Offentliche Gesundheitswesen* 33:681; *Israeli Journal of Medical Science*. 1971. 1209; Seltzer, H. S. 1972. *Diabetes* 21:955–966.

12. Miller, M. 1974. *Competitive Problems in the Drug Industry*. Senate Select Committee on Small Business, Monopoly Subcommittee Hearings, part 25, p. 10801.

13. ____. *Competitive Problems in the Drug Industry*, p. 10801.

14. *Hearings before the Select Committee on Nutrition and Human Needs of the United States Senate*. June 22, 1977.

15. Bressler, R. N. 1977. *New England Journal of Medicine*. 296(14):787–793.

CHAPTER TWO

Understanding the diabetic disease process

There are two major types of diabetes: juvenile-onset and maturity-onset. While both of these terms seem to imply that only young people have juvenile diabetes and only older people have maturity-type diabetes, this is not true. The major differences involve the character of the disease and the way its symptoms are first expressed. In juvenile-onset diabetes the symptoms come on very dramatically and rapidly because the pancreas is producing little or no insulin. These symptoms usually include: 1. frequent urination (polyuria); 2. extreme thirst (polydipsia); 3. ravenous appetite and hunger (polyphagia); 4. weight loss; 5. extreme fatigue; 6. ketoacidosis. Ketoacidosis is the complication that most threatens the juvenile-onset diabetic. It can occur almost anytime in his life. Due to an extreme deficiency of insulin, the patient's blood sugar increases, and his body usually loses tremendous amounts of fluid. The juvenile-onset diabetic then becomes extremely dehydrated, and a dangerous acid condition in his blood develops. If this degenerative process continues without treatment, in extreme cases, or when sufficient insulin and fluids are not administered soon enough, coma and unconsciousness often occur. In order to avoid these potentially death-dealing complications, the juvenile-onset diabetic will probably have to give himself insulin shots for the remainder of his life, and, unfortunately, the rest of his life may not be as long as most people's lives.

Juvenile-onset diabetes is the most severe type of diabetes, and is much less common than the other type. Only about one million of the nation's ten to twenty million known or unknown diabetics have this form of the disease. Physicians can usually recognize it immediately, and as a rule the first thing they do is test the person's urine for sugar. The patient's blood glucose level is usually abnormally high, and can be as high as 1,000 mg (one gram) per 100 ml of blood. The normal blood sugar concentration should be from 65 to 120 mg per 100 ml blood, with 70 mg to 110 mg per 100 ml blood usually considered normal.

The first convincing evidence that juvenile-onset diabetes in humans can be caused by a virus has been reported by investigators from the National Institute of Dental Research (NIDR) and the National Naval Medical Center (NNMC). They isolated a virus known as Coxsackie-B4 from a child who developed diabetes and died within days after the onset of this viral infection; they then demonstrated that this same virus in human pancreas cells infects and damages cultured animals' pancreas cells and induces diabetes in susceptible mice. This discovery suggests that viruses may be involved in the etiology of juvenile-onset diabetes. The most likely viral candidates include the mumps virus, the rubella virus, and members of the Coxsackie virus family. This last group are common, small, RNA containing viruses that can produce upper respiratory infections, muscle pain, and infections of the heart and brain.

An article in *Science* tells the story of this new and exciting research being done at the National Institute of Dental Research:

Within the past year, Notkins and his colleagues have reported that they have been able to demonstrate damage to cultured B cells— those cells in the pancreas that produce insulin—by infection with mumps and Coxsackie B3 viruses. They have also been able to induce diabetes in susceptible mice with type 3 and Coxsackie B4 virus. All four are common infectious agents in humans. They achieved this result by passing each virus many times through cultured B cells. This repeated passaging selects four variants of the virus that replicate readily in the cells and damage them. They also examined different types of mice until they found strains that were susceptible to the viral effects. These results provided a very strong suggestion that viruses play a role in the induction of juvenile-onset diabetes. The most recent findings provide proof.

The new virus specimen was obtained from a previously healthy ten-year-old boy who was admitted to the National Naval Medical Center in a diabetic coma within three days after the onset of symptoms of a flu-like illness. The boy died seven days later and a post mortem examination showed destruction of B cells. Marshall Austin of the National Naval Medical Center contacted Dr. Notkins and his colleagues and provided them with tissue specimens and blood samples from the youth. Inoculation of ground pancreas tissue from the youth into cultures of mouse, monkey, and human cells led to isolation of a virus identified as a variant of Coxsackie B4. Injection of this new virus into susceptible mice produced diabetes, and the investigators were subsequently able to recover the virus from the diabetic.[1]

If the final outcome of this new research indicates that Coxsackie B4 alone or in conjunction with one or more other viruses plays a role in the initiation of diabetes, and in particular, juvenile-onset diabetes, it may well be possible to develop a vaccine against one or more of these viruses and sharply reduce the number of individuals who might contract the disease in the future. Many questions, however, remain to be answered about the precise nature of the juvenile-onset diabetes process. Investigators, for example, have shown that antibodies to Coxsackie B4 virus are present in about half the population. Antibodies to mumps, rubella, and other viruses are also quite common. The obvious question remains why certain individuals are susceptible to these types of infectious invasion while others are not. Moreover, many juvenile-onset diabetics show no evidence of ever having been infected with Coxsackie B4. So we must conclude that there is apparently a multiplicity of causes, some of which are yet unknown, for the disease juvenile-onset diabetes.

Based on the preceding evidence, it seems fair to assert that, in the juvenile-onset diabetic disease process, infectious invasion does play a certain role. But it also seems clear that a true explanation of juvenile-onset diabetes requires more than just a single virus infection theory. As we shall see in subsequent chapters, there are always other metabolic, nutritional and ecologic factors involved in any form of the diabetic disease process. Obviously, since most diabetics survive just long enough to suffer from blindness, gangrene, kidney failure, neuropathy or cardiovascular disease, we must always strive to fight our way out of the one disease-one cause type of thinking.

The most common type of diabetes, usually afflicting up to 90 percent of all diabetics, is maturity-onset. The patients afflicted with this particular type of diabetes are not prone to ketoacidosis, and for that reason do not usually require insulin injections. The maturity-onset diabetic is most distinguishable from the juvenile-onset diabetic by the fact that the illness appears gradually rather than suddenly. The patient usually acquires the disease somewhat later in his life, though he is apt to mimic the juvenile-onset diabetic symptomatic complaints of weakness and dizziness, excessive appetite, indigestion, and a tendency for frequent urination. "The maturity-onset diabetic," writes Dr. Bertrand E. Lowenstein, "is not as sick as is the insulin-requiring diabetic, but he may well develop, although more slowly, the same complications, including retinal disease leading to an accumulation of blind spots, slowness from recovering from infection, especially in the feet and lower legs, kidney disease, problems involving nerve endings in the extremities, and a sixfold higher risk of heart attacks and strokes than has the non-diabetic population."[2] The discovery of maturity-onset type of diabetes usually occurs after the age of forty, although there are a small but significant number of younger persons, some even under the age of twenty, who are found on routine testing to have this type of disease. Satisfactory control of this type of diabetes requires that the patient cooperate with a well-planned program of treatment.

In order to understand the fundamental factors involved in the diabetic disease process, we must appreciate first that the pancreas is the first endocrine-exocrine organ to be influenced by the ecologic contact with ingested foods and/or chemicals. As such we can also well understand the predisposition of the pancreas as the primary shock organ to ingested foods and/or chemicals. This means that the pancreas has the monumental task of making useful metabolic products from the ingested foods and chemicals and also of buffering against reactions to foods and chemicals. An overstimulated pancreas follows the same general law that other overstimulated tissues and organ systems follow, namely, that overstimulation eventually leads to inhibition of function. It is well documented that addiction to alcohol leads to pancreatic insufficiency. What has been little appreciated in the past is that all addictions, be they food, chemical or otherwise, lead to pancreatic insufficiency of varying degrees.

In 1970, on the advice of Sal Klotz, M.D., I (W.P.) read a book entitled *Food Allergy*, by Rinkel, Randolph and Zeller. This book claims that after four days of fasting, foods and chemicals could be clinically assessed on an induction test basis, with symptoms of all kinds disappearing during a period of four days of avoidance, and reappearing when tested with meals of single foods or with chemicals. Headaches, depression, insomnia, tension, and sometimes even hallucinations, delusions and paranoia were described as having been observed during clinical induction food testing.[3]

Herbert Rinkel, M.D., the senior author of *Food Allergy*, had a personal experience which led him to examine closely the possibilities of symptom formation due to foods. At the allergy clinic some of the staff had prepared him a birthday cake. Within a few minutes of eating a piece of it, he fell to the floor, unconscious. When he came to, he was asking the question: "What happened?" He was curious enough to assess the contents of the angel food cake, and discovered that the only food it contained which he had not eaten the past four days was eggs. He usually ate at least an egg a day, because his parents lived on a farm and supplied him with free eggs; however, he had run out of eggs four days before. He discovered that he was able to reproduce the unconscious state he had experienced by avoiding eggs for four days and then allowing himself a single exposure. This experience led him to examine the relationship of food to symptoms of all kinds in all of his patients. After reading an abundance of literature by such medical researchers as Randolph, Mandell, Rinkel and Alvarez[4] I began questioning whether all these doctors could be wrong about what they were saying concerning food reactions and symptom formation. I soon developed the conviction that I too should take these reactions into account in my diagnosis and let the evidence, rather than prejudice, speak for itself. It became evident to me that medicine at large has been negligent about examining the ecologic organic evidence of food and chemical allergies or allergic-like reactions as causes of both physical and mental illness. In fact, broad spectrum ecologic allergy examinations are not even taught to doctors in medical school. I further began to realize that there needs to be added to the patient's history a physical examination and laboratory diagnosis and a broad spectrum ecologic diagnosis: i.e., the patient as he or she is, defective or otherwise, reacting to his or her total environment. Now, I thought, we have available a method by which we as scientists may watch the symptoms leave by avoidance and emerge on exposure. We are, therefore, in a position to engage less in guesswork and more in immediate clinical diagnosis and management of specific allergic reactions.

Having accepted the fact that specific foods may indeed cause certain symptoms (physical and/or mental) in suscepti- ble individuals, what has all this to do with the dangerous shifts in proper blood sugar levels that the diabetic experiences daily in his life? To answer this question, we

must understand that for many years there has existed in
medicine a generalization relating to carbohydrate intolerance. The diabetic (high blood sugar) and the hypoglycemic (low blood sugar) are said to have carbohydrate
intolerance because of the fact that a single carbohydrate
(corn sugar) food test with blood sugar levels monitored
before and after the test meal consistently offers evidence
that a patient cannot properly handle sugar. In view of such
attitudes, it is an obvious conclusion to state that the
blood sugar is either too high or too low because of
carbohydrate intolerance. From this evidence it is also
assumed that all other carbohydrates will not be tolerated.
This reasoning would logically lead to the conclusion
that treatment of these carbohydrate intolerant conditions
(diabetes mellitus and hypoglycemia) consists of reducing
all carbohydrate (especially free carbohydrates) intake by
the patient.

Be this as it may, there are other physicians who have
discovered that hypoglycemia and hyperglycemia (diabetes) can be evoked in a person who has ingested any food or
has come in contact with any chemical to which he is
maladaptively reactive. Broad spectrum food and chemical
symptom induction testing with blood sugar and pH
monitored before and after the test meals reveals the
surprising evidence that low and high blood sugar can be
evoked by foods of all types, whether fat, carbohydrates or
proteins, and that chemicals such as petrochemical
hydrocarbons and even tobacco equally evoke abnormal sugar
level curves in susceptible people. The foods causing these
reactions are specific for each person. Carbohydrates
predominate as symptom precipitating substances, but the
reactions are not limited to carbohydrates. These reactions can
be caused by any substance to which the person reacts
maladaptively. The simple fact of the matter is that abnormal
sugar levels in the body are caused by specific allergic-like
reactions to specific substances. The central problem in
hypoglycemia and diabetes is not, therefore, that of a general
type of food(i.e., carbohydrate), but that of an individual
maladaptive reaction to a specific food or chemical which in

turn interferes with proper blood sugar levels. These maladaptive reactions must always be individually diagnosed
for each person by provocative food testing. Surprisingly
enough, clinical evidence has demonstrated both high
and/or low blood sugar in response to pasteurized cow's
milk, cream cheese, hydrocarbons and many other noncarbo-
hydrate substances. This is not to say that milk will cause
low or high blood sugar in all people, but it does point to
the fact that hypoglycemia as well as hyperglycemia (diabetes) should not be considered strictly in terms of a
carbohydrate metabolism dysfunction. Rather, clinically suspected incriminating substances of all kinds must be seen
in the light of evoked abnormal biochemical individuality
and treated accordingly.

As a psychiatrist I wanted to test clinically the assumption that disordered carbohydrate reactions, whether they
are hypoglycemia or hyperglycemia, are not always a response to carbohydrates alone. One case that clearly
represents this fact was a thirty-year-old man who presented
himself to me for treatment. He had had manic-depressive
reactions in the past; these reactions included psychotic
degrees of depression, a suicide attempt, and dissociated
episodes during which he went places and did things of
which he had no memory. As an infant he was diagnosed as
having a milk allergy and of necessity used soy milk
instead of cow's milk. As an adult he assumed he had
outgrown his milk allergy and daily used dairy products
in large quantities. He was symptom-free by the fourth day
of the fast, using nonchemically treated water only.
A test meal of pasteurized cow's milk plunged him into
the depths of depression. Blood sugar then was normal
before and after the test. With Swiss cheese he was cold
and sweaty. Dairy butter evoked a severe depression. Cream
cheese was a favorite food which he frequently used. He
loved and frequently ate a blue cheese dressing containing
cream cheese. Before the test for cream cheese began, he
was symptom-free. Within fifteen minutes after the test meal
for cream cheese, symptoms began to develop. At first he
felt like withdrawing from other people due to a contempla-

tive and depressive feeling. Within another fifteen minutes
he was severely depressed and withdrew from the hospital
parlor to the seclusion of his room. He reacted overly to
sounds and sights and would cringe as if afraid of being
attacked. At this point, half an hour after the test meal, he
was disassociated and had no memory of what happened
around him. His pulse was 123 fluctuating to 50 and his
blood pressure was 170/110. *At this point his blood sugar
was 20 mg percent.* It was difficult to believe this
and so the test was run four times. Then he was given
specific nutrients: vitamin C, vitamin B6, calcium gluconate, magnesium sulphate, and others which will be discussed in later chapters. With this he awakened, was
communicative, understood, and was not frightened by
environmental stimuli. However, he was too weak to
stand. He also had a pounding headache. His pulse was 80
and blood pressure was 130/84. He was given a dose
of sodium bicarbonate intravenously and his headache
left. He was still too weak to stand, and complained of
spots in his eyes and indistinct vision. His blood sugar
was again taken and found to be only 30 mg percent.
Normal blood sugar would range between 120 mg percent
and 160 mg percent. He was given six teaspoons of beet
sugar, a glass of pineapple juice and several bites of
chocolate cake. Prior testing had demonstrated him not to
be symptom reactive to beet, pineapple, or cereal grains.
Within thirty minutes his blood sugar was a normal 140
mg percent and he was symptom-free other than a slight
apprehension for several hours that the symptom state
could suddenly return.

The low blood sugar attack described above occurring
in response to a food test is the most severe and prolonged
ever observed in our clinic. In this particular case the
assumption that disordered carbohydrate reactions will be
in response to carbohydrates alone is not valid. Testing
reveals that they occur to any type of food and that the
central cause is that of being maladaptively reactive in a
specific way to a certain food (fat, protein, carbohydrate) or
chemical. In the previously mentioned case the hypoglycemic

response was to cream cheese, which is largely a protein and fat food.

A similar yet distinctively different type of food induced maladaptive reaction can also cause diabetes. A forty-five-year-old man, for example, had a morning fasting blood sugar of 250 mg percent. He had already been studied by an allergist and his food and chemical allergies were known. His diabetes mellitus (hyperglycemia) potential had not been assessed, however, since this is not a routine type of analysis in allergy testing. Foods that he had not eaten for several days were chosen for testing until his fasting blood sugar was normal. This required sixteen hours of fasting. He was symptom-free before a test meal, with his blood sugar at 80 mg percent. Forty-five minutes after a test meal with beef his blood sugar soared to 280 mg percent. His symptoms were described as a spaced out feeling, and a sense of a loss of balance when he walked. In this case, a protein food (beef) caused a severe diabetic reaction.

As judged from a study of amino acid metabolism disorders in physical and mental degenerative diseases, we have concluded that brief bouts of hyperammonemia are quite common in degenerative diseases. Sniff test exposures to ammonia reveals that it often evokes symptoms classic of the patient's complaints. The brain is highly sensitive to ammonia and is known to produce anything from minor to major central nervous system reactions in response to hyperammonemia. Muscular weakness is characteristic of hyperammonemia. The extremes of ammonia encephalopathy are found in diabetic ketoadicosis and hepatic coma. It is of special interest to note that hyperammonemia is characteristic of the diabetic disease process.

In infants and children who have failed to thrive, it is sometimes discovered that there is present a hyperammonemia based on specific isolable enzyme deficiencies. The suggestion is strong that disorders such as schizophrenia, manic depressive and psychotic depression likely involve genetic enzyme disorders similar to but of less intensity than the children who failed to thrive due to disordered urea cycle metabolism. Furthermore, others have recently considered the possible significance of episodic hyperammonemia in disordering brain function.

The mental function of inherited protein intolerance due to reduced ornithine transcarbamoylase deficiency on reduced mental capacity was compared with relatives who were not carriers of this disorder.[6] Among the relatives were numerous spontaneous aborters and infant deaths. Matthysse[7] considers that we would do well to be examining mental patients after this model of inherited urea cycle disorder.

There are nine known mechanisms of producing hyperammonemia; five dealing with disordered enzyme function of the urea cycle and four dealing with disordered enzyme function of lysine metabolism. All of these disorders have been observed selectively in mental and physical degenerative diseases and multiples of these existing in a high percentage of cases. It seems evident that addiction evokes enzyme dysfunctions comparable to genetic disorders. When genetic disorders exist, they step up the degenerative disease process and create a state of vulnerability for the development of addiction and a similar maladaptive reactivity to environmental substances. Also, it is observed that the process of degenerative disease evoked by addiction as well as genetic enzyme disorders evoke nutritional deficiencies by the process of excessive demand. Therefore, it is observed that nutritional deficiencies in vitamins, minerals and amino acids frequently exist irrespective of nutritional intake of adequacy or inadequacy.

Metabolic acidosis is observed to emerge during addictive withdrawal, acute maladaptive reactions (to foods, chemicals and inhalants), diabetes and infections. Many body enzyme functions are dependent on a narrow pH range. Metabolic acidosis (1) reduces enzyme function of the urea cycle with the consequences of emerging blood ammonia, (2) produces opiate alkaloids, (3) activates kinin and prostaglandin inflammatory reactions and (4) probably is one of the metabolic disordered conditions necessary for the pathological production of ascorbic acid change to dehydroascorbic acid in the blood.

An overstress of acid-base homeostasis by exclusive use of a single food can in part explain the toxicity of pure foods.[8] Watson[9] documented the therapeutic value of using food sources to maintain an optimum acid-base balance. Randolph[10] documented the therapeutic value of using sodium and potassium bicarbonate to reduce provocatively evoked symptoms. Guinea pigs and humans chronically fed a high acid producing food (wheat) increased dehydro-ascorbic acid with the emergence of a parallel hyperglycemia while at the same time revealing a corresponding lowering of ascorbic acid.[11] When the high wheat diet was fortified with 15 percent casein, the increased dehydroascorbic acid formation and hyperglycemia did not occur. Infections (also acidic evoking) increase dehydroascorbic acid and decrease ascorbic acid. My observations are that acute maladaptive reactions and addictive withdrawal evoke acidic states and are observed to decrease the amount of ascorbic acid. This measured decrease of ascorbic acid in these conditions presumably can be used as an indirect method of measuring an increase in dehydro-ascorbic acid. This needs further clarification.

The conversion of dehydroascorbic acid to ascorbic acid by homocystine[12] requires a pH of 6-8. Conversion of ascorbic acid to dehydroascorbic acid would be antici-pated as requiring an acid medium as one of the necessary conditions. The observed increase in dehydroascorbic acid in acidic states, as well as the decrease of ascorbic acid in these same states, indirectly confirms the likely validity of this assumption. This likelihood is in need of experimental clarification.

Another probable significance of disordered acid-base balance stems from evidence of disordered behavior origi-nating in an imbalance between α-endorphins and γ-endorphins in which an alkaline state is necessary for the production of [des-Tyr] γ-endorphin[13] α-endorphin evokes obsessive-compulsive and stereotyped behavior with an associated reduced ability of response extinction while γ-endorphin provides for the extinction of responses to occur. Thus, it prevents or corrects the development of obsessions, compulsions and stereotyped behavior. It seems likely that the acidic state characteristic of addiction and maladaptive reactions to environmental substances is one of the conditions under which obsessive-compulsiveness, tension and build-up of symptoms occur due to the loss of symptom extinguishability. Another factor is the availability of nutritional precursors necessary for [des-Tyr] γ-endorphins which are tyrosine and leucine. These are frequently deficient due to less than optimum proteolysis from reduced production of pancreatic proteases.

Dehydroascorbic acid and dehydroascorbic are in equilibrium. Most authors refer to this collectively as dehydroascorbic acid. At the cell membrane level, dehydroascorbic serves the purpose of transport through the cell membrane and is reduced to ascorbic acid within the cell.[14] We are concerned with disordered metabolic states that interfere with this normal function of dehydroascorbic for varied reasons causing a rise in serum dehydroascorbic with resultant toxicity.

There is reason to believe that elevated dehydroascorbic[14] exerts a number of toxic effects including autonomic dysfunction, slowed cell division, lymphocytolysis and thymic involution, lipid peroxidation, complexing with SH groups and ascorbic acid-dehydroascorbic redox potential shift in the oxidative direction.[15]

In infectious diseases, blood ascorbic acid decreases and dehydroascorbic acid increases.[16] Pharmacological doses of dehydroascorbic acid are reported to be diabetogenic.[17] Animal experiments indicate large doses of dehydroascorbic acid degenerate the Beta cells of the pancreas.[18,19] Serum dehydroascorbic acid is reported to be continuously elevated in patients with diabetes mellitus.[11] Fetal malformations in diabetes[20] likely result from hyperglycemia interfering with ascorbic acid-dehydroascorbic acid cellular homeostasis.[21] A likely formulation is that addiction and associated infections disorder the metabolic handling of ascorbic acid and dehydroascorbic acid in which the disordered state of metabolism oxidizes ascorbic acid to dehydroascorbic acid which then adversely effects pancreatic Beta cells and many other body functions including central nervous system functions (not as yet assessed).

In addiction to non-narcotic substances the body evokes its own addictive narcotics (methionine-enkephalin, leu-enkephalin, opioid alkaloids) out of its disordered metabolism. These self-produced narcotics are as equally addicting as externally supplied narcotics.[22] The brain and the gut contain the same receptor sites for narcotics. Therefore, we have both central nervous system and gut disordered function, including that of the pancreas, from self-evoked endorphins. Exorphins from partially digested proteins producing long chain peptides of opiate value also influence the central nervous system and pancreas. Therefore, it can be understood how addiction with its production of both endorphins and exorphins is one of the mechanisms helping to produce diabetes.

More case histories revealing allergically induced diabetes

Carl is a fifteen-year-old boy diagnosed as a juvenile-onset diabetic by two physicians. He was receiving insulin when he came to my clinic in November 1978. Upon examining him, it was noted that he consumed great amounts of dairy products, cereal grains, potatoes, grapes and apples. When placed on infrequently used foods (given sometimes as a substitute method of fasting) he did not manifest his usual rise in blood sugar, and ketones cleared in his urine. It was soon evident that he was a maturity-onset diabetic and not insulin dependent. Upon testing him for maladaptive reactions, he was found to be a very serious reactor to cereal grains and dairy products. Both wheat and oats as well as milk produced hyperglycemia reactions well above 230 mg percent. His long-standing symptom of lethargy was also evoked by wheat and his frequent headaches were evoked by oats.

I have observed for quite some time many diabetics who reacted very seriously to petrochemical hydrocarbons such as found in exhaust fumes from cars, in perfumes, or in fumes from natural gas. In Carl's case, a thirty minute test exposure to auto exhaust, as is usually experienced in city traffic, produced a shift in blood sugar from 90 mg percent before exposure to well over 180 mg percent after the exposure.

Carl does not just have diabetes; as with most diabetics, he has other symptoms such as weakness, headaches, irritability, depression, and so forth. These reactions are part and parcel of an allergic-like-addictive syndrome to specific foods and chemicals, and are not in themselves evidence of a psychological illness due to psychological causes. His headaches and feelings of weakness, for example, have already been clinically demonstrated to be reactions to foods and chemicals.

Another example of an maladaptively reactive chemical diabetic state is offered to us by a thirty-eight-year-old chronic undifferentiated schizophrenic of fifteen years' duration. The patient presented symptoms of social withdrawal, hostility, apathy, apprehension, depression and obsessional thinking. There was marked improvement by the fourth day of the fast on distilled water only. Deliberate food testing with one hundred and fifteen different foods revealed symptom reactions to forty-three foods. There was a hyperglycemia (diabetic) reaction with symptoms to eight foods, and hyperglycemia reactions alone to three foods. Six hyperglycemia responses were beyond 200 mg percent with the highest being cane sugar at 210 mg percent. The protein food of whole milk produced hyperglycemia of 200 mg percent at one hour after the meal, while the high carbohydrate foods maple syrup and honey produced normal ranges of only 135 mg percent and 110 mg percent respectively. Symptoms associated with hyperglycemia reaction evoked during the test were a marked apprehension, obsessional thoughts, sleepiness, a feeling of being high, weakness, tiredness and stomach cramps.

Another example of a maladaptively induced diabetic

reaction is given to us by a fifty-four-year-old Mexican
woman diagnosed as a diabetic four years before she came
to our clinic. Diet and insulin management were used by
other physicians for her complications. She was difficult to
manage, and was hospitalized twice a year in the four
years prior to her coming to the clinic. During the
hospitalization she usually had blood sugars of 400 mg
percent or worse. Her presenting symptoms were marked
weakness, blurred vision and severe depression. When she
came to our clinic she was placed on a fast of distilled
water only. Food testing was started on the fifth day and
by that day her strength had returned, her vision was normal
and her depression was gone. Blood sugar was taken
before and one hour after each test meal. Blood sugar was
monitored with the Eye-tone meter. She was tested for
forty-three foods, twenty-nine of which produced either
symptoms or hyperglycemia (diabetes) beyond 160 mg
percent. Six foods evoked hyperglycemia without associated
symptoms, while twenty-three foods evoked both hyperglycemia and associated symptoms. The highest blood sugar
reading was for rice at 340 mg percent, and the next was
sweet potatoes at 320 mg percent. Fifteen foods had readings of 200 mg percent and beyond. Tuna, a protein food,
produced a blood sugar of 300 mg percent; pinto beans gave
a reading of 190 mg percent; and spinach proved out at
190 mg percent. On the other hand, maple syrup produced a
normal reading of only 120 mg percent with no symptoms;
oranges as well as pears both produced a reading of 130 mg
percent with no symptoms.

It was thus observed that there were infrequently used
carbohydrates that caused neither symptoms nor a hyperglycemic reaction, while there were also frequently used
proteins that did in fact cause both symptoms and hyperglycemia. The cereal grains of rice, millet, mature corn, oats,
rye and wheat all evoked symptoms with blood sugars
ranging up from 200 mg percent. Interestingly enough,
however, maple syrup, which our clinic's patient had
never eaten before, produced a blood sugar of only 120 mg

percent (normal). Normal post test meal blood sugars are less than 160 mg percent.

A case of a nonfood maladaptive reaction induced diabetic state is exemplified to us by a twenty-five-year-old man who was observed to be delusional and had compulsive verbalizing during his delusions after smoking a cigarette. He was also excessively hungry and thirsty most of the time. His morning fasting blood sugars were erratic, usually ranging between 100 mg percent and 150 mg percent, but on several occasions there were ranges exceeding 200–250 mg percent. It was discovered that when his fasting blood sugars were abnormally high, he was sneaking a cigarette before the test. We then decided to test this young man's sugar levels while he was smoking. He was not allowed to smoke a cigarette for four days. His fasting sugar was 75 mg percent and he was symptom-free before the test. He smoked eight cigarettes in thirty minutes. During the test he became delusional and compulsively verbalized his delusions, starting with the second cigarette. At thirty minutes after starting the smoking test his blood sugar soared to over 200 mg percent (hyperglycemia).

A twenty-four-year-old man was a three pack a day cigarette smoker. He went twenty-four hours without smoking before a cigarette smoking test. His blood sugar was 80 mg percent before the test. With the first cigarette he was sweating and too weak to stand. At thirty minutes after the test began his blood sugar dropped to 30 mg percent (severe hypoglycemia).

Based on the previous examples, as well as hundreds of other case histories at our clinic, it is obvious that both hypoglycemia and hyperglycemia can be evoked by maladaptive reactions to all forms of food as well as tobacco. The cases cited above offer convincing evidence of this fact. It has also been observed clinically that petrochemical hydrocarbons such as exhaust fumes, perfumes, gas stoves or heating units are equally potent sources in producing a disordered carbohydrate metabolism.

We shall conclude our discussion at this point by asserting that an ecologic-metabolic diagnosis of diabetes mellitus reveals diabetic reactions to carbohydrates as well as fats, proteins and chemicals. It equally reveals carbohydrates, fats, proteins and chemicals to which there are no symptoms and diabetic reactions on exposure. As such, only specific substances reacted to that evoke insulin resistance or inhibit pancreatic production of insulin and pancreatic function as a whole are capable of producing abnormal carbohydrate metabolism. This, of course, means that the concept of carbohydrate interference being caused by many different yet specific substances is more characteristic of diabetes mellitus than the narrow view that diabetes mellitus is a singular metabolic entity caused by a general carbohydrate intolerance. The stress building blocks of diabetes mellitus therefore can only be determined by a broad spectrum ecologic-metabolic food maladaptive reactive diagnosis and cannot be accurately diagnosed by the single food (corn) glucose tolerance test.

Hans Selye taught us that chronic stress, physical or emotional, leads to chronic illness, physical or emotional. Of all the many stresses that plague mankind, the linked ones of allergic-like maladaptive and addictive reactions are of the greatest intensity and most prolonged, and therefore are frequently central causes of physical or emotional symptoms, either temporary or chronic. The extent and nature of such stresses vary markedly from person to person. Each individual's ability to handle toxins, pollens, and foods and chemicals contacted from the environment differs considerably, according to his unique chemical makeup. The more defective this individual biochemical makeup is, by inheritance, enzyme deficiency, malnutrition, harbored infection or otherwise, the more likely the person is to develop maladaptive allergic-like symptoms on exposure to food and environmental contacts. Our peculiar cultural preferences for eating only a few types of food, for example, or our heavy consumption of refined carbohydrates, or the chronic use of alcohol and tobacco, add materially to a developing state of nutritional deficiency with a corresponding multiple symptom production in our body tissue systems. Likewise, our nation's propensity to consume nutritionally deficient junk foods further increases the defective tissue states in the human body. These defective tissue states undermine an individual's ability to handle without symptom formation the contacts he has with toxins, pollens, foods or chemical fumes. Whether we call these reactions allergic (immunologic) or allergic-like (nonimmunologic) is immaterial. The significant facts are: 1. reactions by symptom formation occur between the relatively intact human organisms and their environmental contact; 2. these reactions are consistent and therefore reproducible by anyone who follows the known rules for evoking symptoms; 3. the greater the defectiveness of the organism, the greater the likelihood of such maladaptive reactions occurring. In our clinic, biochemical monitoring reveals that maladaptive reactions, such as the chronic addiction reactions and their counterpart allergic reactions to foods, chemicals and inhalants, are the central stress building blocks from which many degenerative diseases are constructed. Diabetes mellitus, obviously, is one of these degenerative diseases. The chronic physical and mental reactions described in the preceding case histories were observed to fade in intensity, and often to disappear completely, on a four to six day fast or period of infrequently used foods and with complete avoidance of chemicals; they then acutely emerged again on exposure to test meals of food or chemicals of different kinds. These reactions provide impressive evidence of having actually, under controlled experimental conditions, turned off an illness while knowing why, and of having turned the illness on again and knowing why. But the question remains: what relationship does a period of four to six days have to an allergic reaction? Why should the avoidance of a chemical or a certain food for a specific period result in a severe hyperglycemic symptom when a sensitive person is exposed to that chemical or food after the period of avoidance? The answers to these questions and others lie in a proper understanding of addiction and maladaptive allergic-like reactions.

Addiction is described as a state involving withdrawal phase symptoms of any kind occurring hours or days (up to three days) after contact with a particular substance. Similarly, these withdrawal phase symptoms can often be stopped—sometimes only partially—by continued contact with the addictive substance. Foods of all kinds as well as chemicals qualify as much as do narcotics, tobacco, coffee and alcohol. But for our purposes of explanation, tobacco addiction can be cited as a model. Since about 75 percent of all humans are maladaptively symptom reactive to tobacco, their first contact occasions immediate allergic-like symptoms: most usually experience nausea, dizziness and/or a cough. With frequent use, these symptoms are suppressed by the tobacco contact, and later emerge, if there is no continued use of tobacco, as withdrawal symptoms. These symptoms can be kept suppressed only if the tobacco is contacted frequently enough to keep the user in a relief or postponed state. This state of partial and temporary relief by contact with the allergen is termed addiction. Understanding addiction as an extension of a maladaptive allergic-like state is necessary if one is to understand the seriousness of the addiction to frequently eaten foods and commonly met chemicals which plagues about 80 percent of mankind.

Adaptive addiction can be described as a state of relative freedom from symptoms, occasioned when the addictive substance is contacted frequently enough and the biological homeostatic state is in good repair. It is, however, a state of chronic stress, precariously balanced, and paves the way for the emergence of an "illness"—an acute allergic reaction previously described—upon the addition of stress of any kind. Such last straw stresses may be: 1. an overload of the allergen or otherwise maladaptive reactive substance; 2. the addition of seasonal allergens such as pollens or other environmental stress; 3. physical stresses such as excessive cold, heat or fatigue; 4. harbored infections; 5. emotional stress. The person suffering from adaptive addiction may be likened to one walking a tightrope, from which he may easily fall at any time. If the patient

falls from the tightrope—that is, develops an illness—
solving that immediate stress, physiological or psychological,
merely restores him to the adaptive-addictive tightrope,
leaving him the prey of any wind of stress that blows into
his life. However, if the basic addiction is handled, he then
has a broad base from which to handle all stress—he is on
firm ground, so to speak, and off the tightrope. It is in this
sort of situation that we psychiatrists so frequently give
only a partial answer to our patients' needs—tranquilizers,
antidepressants, and the like— solving a little conflict here
and there but failing to solve the basic underlying metabolic
problem of addiction and other maladaptive reactions to
foods and chemicals.

Dr. Theron G. Randolph has clinically demonstrated
that when there is a break in exposure to addictive substances of any kind for at least four days—it seems to take
at least four days for any food or chemical to be entirely
eliminated from the human system—then the addictive
adaptive reaction is converted to an immediate reaction
with an allergic-like quality upon renewed exposure to the
substance. This is, in fact, not a new discovery: Hippocrates
reports in his writings the knowledge that if a food was
avoided for as much as four days, a reexposure to that food
might create a severe reaction in certain people. And this
point cannot be overemphasized: *all* addictions display this
pattern, whether they are narcotic, alcohol, tobacco, food
or chemical in source. In our clinic, we have observed that
removing the patient for four or more days from contact
with any suspected food or chemical addictive substances
and then selectively reexposing him to one substance at a
time has produced the emergence of every shade of physical
and mental symptom described in medical literature,
including severe shifts in blood sugar levels, plus a host of
common somatic symptoms often classed as psychosomatic.
Such allergic-like maladaptive reactions can either excite or
inhibit any tissues or organs in the body (including the
pancreas), and are, therefore, capable of giving rise to
any set of symptoms these tissues are able to produce.

Further considerations of the four to six day period of avoidance

During the first two or three days of a fast or period of infrequently used foods, symptoms often emerge. This is not caused by a starving need for nutrients, but by the withdrawal phase symptoms of an addiction. A person without food addictions will not display symptoms on a four day period of avoidance.

Usually by the fourth day of avoidance such symptoms will have materially subsided or disappeared. If they have not subsided by the fourth day, the period of avoidance should be extended by one to three days to see if the patient improves. In some of the more severely allergic cases, four days of avoidance are not enough for the symptoms to clear, and can be extended up to seven days. This type of program is indicated for some chronically ill patients. It should be remembered that if there is not adequate environmental control, symptoms may continue because of exposure to a substance (e.g., smoke, gas, hydrocarbon pollution) to which the person is reacting.

Asthmatics, epileptics, diabetics on insulin and markedly debilitated patients should be tested and treated under direct medical supervision. On the withdrawal of food, as well as the reentry of foods at test meals, asthmatic attacks or very severe diabetic reactions can be evoked in susceptible people. Emotional reactions in food sensitive persons during the avoidance period and also during the food testing can range from mild—such as tension, fatigue, headache, dizziness—to marked psychotic and insightless states involving deep depression and a wish to die, hallucinations, delusions and illogical aggression. It is therefore advised that when testing or detoxifying (through fasting or avoidance periods of only infrequently used foods) any markedly debilitated patient, an objective observer be available so that emergency medical help can be obtained if needed. It helps to realize that the symptoms occurring

during the food testing are likely to subside in one to three
hours, although in some cases it may be as much as five
hours, and occasionally reactions have lasted up to three
days. In these more severe cases, medical assistance to stop
the reaction is indicated. The method by which this is
accomplished will be discussed later. However, in most
cases the symptoms will fade in a short time.

Water that is not chemically treated (i.e., spring, well,
distilled or filtered water) is used during testing since
some people are known to react to chlorine and/or fluorine.
There must be no smoking during the period of avoidance
or the subsequent test days. If there are no symptoms by
the fourth day of the avoidance period, tobacco can be
tested if desired. This is achieved by chain-smoking as fast
as possible a maximum of six cigarettes. The test ends as
soon as symptoms develop. Dizziness, nausea and weakness
are common minor symptoms of tobacco allergy, and in
many cases blood sugar levels are dramatically altered for
the worse. If the person will agree to stop smoking without
such a test, this is the better plan. Some people will
remember the symptoms that developed when they smoked
their first cigarette. When they are informed that this is
evidence of allergy to tobacco, that is sufficiently convincing for these people to stop smoking. These are the lucky
ones, for there is always the danger during the tobacco test
of judgment being affected or of aggressive behavior flaring
up. But if the patient has to be convinced that he is
tobacco allergic, then the test must be done.

In any food allergy testing program, a comprehensive
environmental control plan is vital. The purpose of environmental control is to isolate the person from all substances
to which he or she may be reacting: fumes, animal dander,
cosmetics, hair conditioners, perfumes, gas, air pollution
containing industrial waste, dye odors, certain soaps used
for cleaning, oil or gas from furnaces, moth balls, spray
fresheners and so forth. Obviously, it is much easier to
arrange for an adequate environmental control in a hospital setting where a unit has been especially designed for this
purpose; in some cases, this is an absolute necessity. If

during the fourth or fifth day of the fast, the pulse still remains high or there still remain ongoing common symptoms (including hyper- and/or hypoglycemia), then it is probably due to a lack of proper environmental control. In this case the environment must be reexamined to see if there is some agent to which the person is reacting. The pulse should be below 85 before testing. The same withdrawal phase symptoms that occur with food addiction can occur on the second to third day of avoidance of incriminating environmental factors. This fact is important to remember, since in some cases the environmental factor is more the culprit in the patients' illness than their food.

If a person reacts maladaptively to a food when occasionally eaten, he is aware of this, and hence does not like the food. Such reactions to infrequently eaten foods are rare and obviously are not associated with the chronic addictive state. A food has to be eaten two or more times a week to be addicting. The more frequently a food is eaten, the more likely it is to be incriminated in addiction. However, even though a food is infrequently eaten, it may belong to a family of which a member is frequently eaten, such as legumes, squash-melon-cucumber, dairy products and gluten-bearing cereal grains (wheat, rye, oats, barley, corn). One member of a family eaten frequently predisposes a person to maladaptive reactions to other members of the same family, even if infrequently eaten.

A choice has to be made as to the types of food to be tested: 1. foods grown without insecticides; 2. market grown foods which will contain insecticide residues; 3. raw foods; 4. cooked foods; 5. foods with preservatives and colors added. Theoretically, each of these categories needs to be tested separately. Sometimes a food can be eaten raw when it cannot be eaten cooked, or vice-versa. Sometimes foods without spray residues can be eaten without a reaction. Sometimes there are reactions to food colors and preservatives. The most practical way is to start with the food as usually eaten: market grown fruits, vegetables and meats which are either cooked or raw. Definitive testing can then be done on those foods in which reactions occur.

Colors and preservatives are left out of the initial food testing. If more than fifteen foods are reacted to, then insecticide residues should be suspected and several of the reactive foods retested from sources not containing insecticides. Ideally, but difficult to achieve, is the initial testing of basic foods not containing insecticide residues. Some physicians are achieving this goal and for certain patients it is a necessity.

In conclusion, it seems valid to assert, based on clinical evidence and induction testing, that both hypoglycemia and hyperglycemia (diabetes) have the same basic source of allergic-like addiction in the majority of cases. Whether the response is low or high blood sugar depends on the stage of the stress reaction. Hypoglycemia can be characterized as the "adaptation stage" (Hans Selye, *The Stress of Life*) of the stress allergic reaction with the characteristic reaction of hyperinsulinism (too much insulin which causes the sugar levels in the blood to drop); hyperglycemia (diabetes) can be characterized as the "exhaustion stage" of the stress allergic reactions of (1) initial cell membrane insulin resistance in the face of hyperinsulinism, and (2) late stage hypoinsulinism either of which causes the blood sugar to rise. The progression of the development from hypoglycemia to adult-onset diabetes mellitus is suggested in this order: 1. acute allergic-like maladaptive reactions (i.e. essentially addictive) to foods and chemicals, with stress of the addictive and/or similar maladaptive reactions first involving the pancreas (alarm stage); 2. several years of adaptive addictive adjustment with the consequences of episodic hypoglycemia (adaptation stage); 3. metabolic failure by fatigue and/or exhaustion of the adaptation stage resulting in a more complete deterioration of the function of the pancreas and the logical onset of diabetes mellitus (exhaustion stage). The cell membrane disorder resulting in insulin resistance, frequently initially observable in maturity-onset diabetes, is a manifestation of the diabetes mellitus disease process. Insulin resistance is observed to be readily reversible by avoiding the demonstrable maladaptive reactive foods, chemicals and inhalants.

Once chronic addictive reactions and their counterpart acute allergic-like maladaptive reactions to foods, chemicals and inhalants become the central stress factor that produces the pancreatic deficiency disease process known as diabetes mellitus, there are certain very specific metabolic events that occur within the pancreas itself. B. M. Frier, M.D., has given convincing evidence, for example, that diabetes mellitus should by definition encompass a concept of "generalized pancreatic insufficiency."[23] By this he means that in the diabetic state, the pancreas's production of bicarbonate is the most deficient, followed by its secretion of proteolytic enzymes, and last and least of all, by insulin production. After thinking about this idea, it becomes obvious that rather than characterizing diabetes mellitus simply as carbohydrate intolerance caused by the single specific factor of a deficiency in insulin production, as is done by many physicians today, it is more correct to describe the diabetes mellitus disease process as a maladaptive allergic-like addictive stress related disease resulting in an initial excitation causing a later inhibition of *all* the life sustaining functions of the pancreas gland. More specifically, this implies that once the chronic onset of maladaptive responses has inhibited the various functions of the pancreas gland, and has thus caused abnormal blood sugar levels in a particular patient, careful and therapeutic attention must first be directed to that patient's pancreatic production of bicarbonate and proteolytic enzymes, since as our clinical experience will demonstrate, more often than not generalized pancreatic deficiency (diabetes) can be corrected at this level first (i.e., by the removal of the allergic-like-addictive stress factors coupled with the supplementation of bicarbonate and proteolytic enzymes) without the introduction of insulin at all. John Potts, M.D., did a statistical study on bio-ecologic diagnosis and found that two-thirds of the insulin dependent adult-onset diabetics did not need insulin after they had withdrawn from their maladaptive reactive substances. Those still using insulin required only one-third the amount used before their work-up.[24] That's right! Even though you are a diagnosed diabetic currently taking insulin shots, you may in fact not need these daily injections if the proper diagnosis of your food allergies is clinically established and acted upon with a corresponding diet (see Chapter 4) and if supplements of bicarbonate, pancreatic proteolytic enzymes and (as we shall discover in subsequent chapters) a full range of nutrients are all given in therapeutic amounts.

In order for us to see precisely how all these important aspects of treatment fit into the total picture of Ortho-molecular-Ecologic diabetic therapy, let us continue with our discussion by looking at all the vital functions of the pancreas that may be inhibited by the varied stresses of allergic-addictive responses to foods and chemicals.

REFERENCES

1. *Science.* June 15, 1979. 204:4398.

2. Lowenstein, B. E. 1976. *Diabetes.* New York: Harper and Row, p. 10.

3. Rinkel, H. J., et al. 1951. *Food allergy.* Springfield, IL.: Charles C. Thomas.

4. Alvarez, W. C. 1952. *The Neuroses, Diagnosis and Management of Functional Disorders and Minor Psychoses.* Philadelphia: Saunders; Campbell, M. B. 1970. *Allergy of the Nervous System.* Springfield, IL.: Charles C. Thomas; Coca, A. F. 1956. *The Pulse Test.* New York: Arco; Crook, W. G. 1973. Allergy, the great masquerader. *Pediatric Basics.* Gerber; Dees, S. C. 1951. *Allergy in Relation to Pediatrics.* Minneapolis: Bruce; Dickey, L. D. 1976. *Clinical Ecology.* Springfield, IL.: Charles C. Thomas; Frier, B. M. 1976. Exocrine pancreatic function in juvenile-onset diabetes mellitus. *Gut* 17:685–691; Mandell, Marshall. 1970. *Cerebral Reactions in Allergic Patients.* Connecticut: New England Foundation for Allergy; Philpott, W. H. and Kalita, D. K. 1980. *Brain Allergies: The Psychonutrient Connection.* New Canaan, CT.: Keats Publishing; Randolph, T. G. 1953. Food allergy and food addiction. Ninth Annual Congress, American College of Allergists, Chicago; Randolph T. G. 1974. A history of ecologic mental

illness. *Allergy*. Flushing, New York: Medical Examination Publishing, pp. 425–441; Rapaport, H. G. 1970. *The Complete Allergy Guide*. New York: Simon and Schuster; Speer, Frederick, 1970. *Allergy of the Nervous System*. Springfield, IL.: Charles C. Thomas.

5. Pangborn, J.B. and Philpott, W.H. 1981. *Chemical Aspects of Hyperammonemia Observed During Bio-ecologic Diagnosis and Treatment*. Oklahoma City, OK: The Institute for Bio-Ecologic Medicine.

6. Batshaw, M.L., Roan, Y. Jung, A.L., Rosenberg, L.A. and Brusilow, S.W. 1980. Cerebral dysfunction in asymptomatic carriers of ornithine transcarbamylase deficiency. *New England J. Medicine* 302, 9, 482.

7. Matthysse, S. 1980. Genetic detection of cerebral dysfunction. *New England J. of Medicine* 302, 9, 516.

8. Boyd, E.M. 1973. *Toxicity of Pure Foods*. Cleveland: CRC Press.

9. Watson, G. 1972. *Nutrition and Your Mind*. New York: Harper & Row.

10. Randolph, T.G. 1976. The enzymatic, acid, hypoxia, endocrine concept of allergic inflammation. In: *Clinical Ecology*. L.D. Dickey, ed. Springfield, IL.: C.C. Thomas, 577-596.

11. Chatterjee, I.B., Majumber, A.K., Nandi, B.K., et al. 1975. Synthesis and some major functions of vitamin C in animals. *Ann. N.Y. Acad. Sci.* 258:24-47.

12. Hughes. 1956. *Biochem. J.* 64:203-208.

13. De Wied, David 1978. Psychopathology as a Neuropeptide Dysfunction. *Characteristics and Function of Opioids*. J.M. van Ree and L. Terenius, eds. Amsterdam: Elsevier North-Holland Biomedical Press, 113-122.

14. Lewin, S. 1976. *Vitamin C: Its Molecular Biology and Medical Potential*. New York: Academic Press, Figure 1.4.

15. Ely, J.T.A. October 1, 1981. Hyperglycemia and major congenital Anomalies. *N. Engl. J. Med.*

    Ely, J.T.A. 1981. University of Washington, Seattle, WA. Personal communication.

16. Chakrabarti, B. and Banerjee, S. 1955. Dehydroascorbic acid level in blood of patients suffering from various infectious diseases. *Proc. Soc. Exp. Biol. Med.* 88:581-583.

17. Patterson, J.W. 1950. *J. Biol. Chem.* 183:81-88.

18. Massina, A., Brucchieri, A. and Gasso, G. 1968. *Botl. Soc. Ital. Biol. Sper.* 44 (14), 1138-1141.

19. MacDonald, M.K. and Bhattacharya, S.K. 1956. *Quart. J. Exp. Physiol.* 41(2), 153-161.

20. Miller, E., Hare, J.W., Cloherty, J.P., et al. 1981. Elevated maternal hemoglobin A_1C in early pregnancy and major congenital anomalies in infants of diabetic mothers. *New Engl. J. Med.* 304:1331-1334.

21. Mann, G.V. and Newton, P. 1975. The membrane transport of ascorbic acid. *Ann. N.Y. Acad. Sci.* 258:243-252.

    Mann, G.V. 1974. Hypothesis: the role of vitamin C in diabetic angiopathy. *Perspect. Biol. Med.* 4:210-217.

22. Klee, W.A. 1977. Endogenous opiate peptides. In: *Peptides in Neurobiology*, H. Gainer, ed. New York: Plenum Press, 375-396.

23. Frier, B.M. Exocrine pancreatic function in juvenile-onset diabetes mellitus.

24. Potts, John, M.D. and Lang, Melvin S. 1977. Avoidance provocative food testing in assessing diabetes responsiveness. *Diabetes*, vol. 26, supp. 1 #234.

    Potts, J. 1980. Avoidance provocative food testing in assessing diabetes responsiveness. *Diabetes* 29, 6.

    Potts, J.,M.D. 1981. *Diabetes*, Reprint Supplement #1, vol. 30.

CHAPTER THREE

Victory Over Diabetes

Because you are a human being, you have a body whose
structure is both elegant and complex. It is a highly
complicated, dynamic, superbly organized system consisting
of over sixty trillion living cells. Each living cell in your
body is a very unique structure of life. There is no typical or
average cell; different types have distinctive structures,
and each is marvelous in design and organization. The cell
of average size contains about one quadrillion molecules
of different sizes and shapes. Some molecules are hundreds
of times as large as others, and unlike cells, these molecules, though often in rapid motion, are not alive. When the
human body is viewed from a perspective of molecules and
living cells, it is a wonderful, incredible biochemical
machine in which there are literally thousands of chemical
and biochemical reactions taking place every microsecond
of our lives. Each reaction requires certain optimum
conditions in just the right amounts of certain chemical
substances for maximum benefit. Accordingly, as Dr.
Roger Williams has described, each cell is like a factory
complex:

Every cell has its own power from which it derives its energy. The burning process from which energy is derived is a highly ordered, many-step process in which many different catalysts are involved. Each catalyst (enzyme) is protein in nature and is made up of hundreds of amino acids (and often vitamins) put together in exactly the right way. The power plant makes it possible for every cell to be highly dynamic. Something is happening every microsecond. Complex chemical transformations— filtering, ultrafiltering, emulsifying, dispersion, aggregating, absorption—are continually in progress. Tearing down, building up, and repairing are constantly going on.

Cells have their own ways of designing and making blue- prints; "printing" and duplicating are very much in evidence. Cells also have their own versions of assembly lines. They have transportation systems; sorting, pumping, and streaming; and molecules riding piggy-back on others are common processes. Intricate mechanisms, including feedbacks, are used by cells to regulate their numerous activities.

Cells have communication systems—messages and messen- gers. They have the equivalent of both an intercom system and devices for sending and receiving messages to and from the outside. Electrical activities are continually manifest. Cells are equipped with sewage and disposal systems. They even have in effect pollution-control mechanisms whereby toxic molecules are converted into others which are relatively harmless.[1]

In order to achieve optimum health in one's complex physical body, it is first necessary, at least partially, to understand its biochemical functions. Such an understand- ing can be realized by becoming more fully aware of all the important functions of the various glands throughout the body. In the case of our study on diabetes, we should thus direct our attention toward that most vital gland called the pancreas.

The pancreas is one gland among many in the human body and is composed of millions of living cells. It is situated below and behind the stomach. The gland weighs about half a pound, and within the pancreas, especially in the tail, are very small pieces of tissue called the islets of Langerhans. Every normal pancreas has about one hundred thousand or more islets of Langerhans, and each islet contains somewhere between eighty and a hundred beta cells. The beta cells are those structures within the pancreas, first described in 1869, which secrete insulin. Each functioning beta cell is capable of measuring blood glucose levels every ten seconds within the body, and surprisingly enough, to within a range of 2 mg percent accuracy. Within a minute to a minute and a half, these beta cells can organize themselves so as to deliver any amount of insulin necessary to maintain health within the body.

Once the insulin has been released by the beta cells, it has very definite and vital roles to perform in the body. In general terms, it is the main messenger which gives the body signals that control the storage and mobilization of our food and our energy. More specifically, insulin is that hormone that controls the proper levels of blood glucose (blood sugar) throughout the entire system of cells within the human body. The beta cell, when first stimulated by glucose as well as other foods in the diet, releases insulin already stored within itself. As the level of glucose increases in the blood, a signal is sent to the nucleus (or "brain") of the beta cell. This signal is then relayed to the production area of the beta cell and more insulin is produced. If there is any deficiency of insulin production within the beta cells, blood sugar levels continue to increase so that high blood sugar results. This condition is known as diabetes.

The diabetic disease process can also produce a cell membrane disorder resulting in insulin resistance which will cause a rise in blood sugar despite even a hyperinsulinism. An overstressed pancreas due to insulin resistance eventually results in a fatigued inhibition of pancreatic function. These conditions evoking hyperglycemia are known as diabetes mellitus.

From a more technical point of view, the beta cells in the islets of Langerhans first secrete a product known as proinsulin, which is composed of a chain of eighty-one amino acids. This amino acid chain of proinsulin is broken down in an area of the beta cell called the Golgi Apparatus into two chemical substances. The first substance is called insulin but is now a chain of only fifty-one amino acids.

The remaining thirty amino acids are commonly called
C-peptide. Both of these amino acid units of chemical
structure are stored and released when necessary in response to stimulation. The C-peptide structure of proinsulin
has no known effect within the body, but it is released
simultaneously into the circulation of the blood with the
insulin molecule.

As previously mentioned, just as thousands of words
are made from twenty-six letters of our alphabet, so too is
the structure of insulin made from a combination of very
specific amino acids. Amino acids are in reality the founda-
tional building blocks of all life and are the chemical
structures used by the body to construct all the trillions of
living cells contained therein. Of course, not only is
insulin made from a specific combination of amino acids,
but so too are the pancreas and other glands and organs and
life systems in the human body.

The process by which the construction of amino acids
into living cells occurs is a very complicated biochemical
event. When proteins in our food are eaten, the digestive
processes of a healthy individual break them down into
amino acids, which then pass into the blood and are
carried throughout the body. The cells then select the
specific amino acids they need and use them in construct-
ing new body tissues and organs and all such vital substances as antibodies, hormones, enzymes and new blood
cells. If your diet is adequate in protein, your body, with the
help of enzymes and other chemical substances, will
continually make new cells from the building blocks of
amino acids. Amino acids, therefore, are needed continuously from birth until death.

Scientists now tell us that there are basically twenty-two
amino acids, and when isolated, these are white crystalline
substances. Eight of the twenty-two amino acids present in
proteins are growth and maintenance chemicals and, as
such, are absolutely essential constituents of an adequate
diet. These eight amino acids are called essential amino
acids since the body by itself cannot make them. They in
fact must be received from a food source. All the other

fourteen nonessential amino acids can be made by the body cells from fat or sugar combined with nitrogen freed from the breakdown of used proteins. The terms essential and nonessential are a bit misleading since all the twenty-two amino acids are essential to health even though it is not necessary that fourteen of them be acquired from food.

Essential amino acids are supplied in greatest abundance in such foods as egg yolk, fresh milk, kidneys, liver, Brewer's yeast and soybeans; these foods have the highest protein value. Proteins from muscle meats, used in roasts, steaks or chops, are complete but contain fewer of some essential amino acids than do glandular meats. A list of the twenty-two amino acids accompanied by their chemical structure is contained in Figure 3.1.

Diabetes and the pancreas

The proper maintenance of constant and adequate glucose (blood sugar) levels in the body is one of the most important functions of our biochemical being. Your brain needs glucose in order to think clearly; your muscles need glucose for strength and action; in fact your entire body needs glucose to maintain life. A delicately regulated process of the body insures that we have proper levels of glucose in our blood. The anterior pituitary gland which produces hormones that elevate blood sugar, the adrenal medulla which produces epinephrine (adrenaline) that stimulates the breakdown of stored glycogen (carbohydrate stored in the liver), and the adrenal cortex, which produces a number of hormones called glucosteroids that are necessary for the metabolism of all carbohydrates, simultaneously act like instruments in a harmonious and complex symphony of metabolism just so that an adequate level of glucose can be supplied to the body.

When an individual eats a food, it is broken down or digested and then absorbed chiefly as sugar into the bloodstream. In other words, eating food increases blood

FIGURE 3.1:

Eight Essential Amino Acids

Phenylalanine

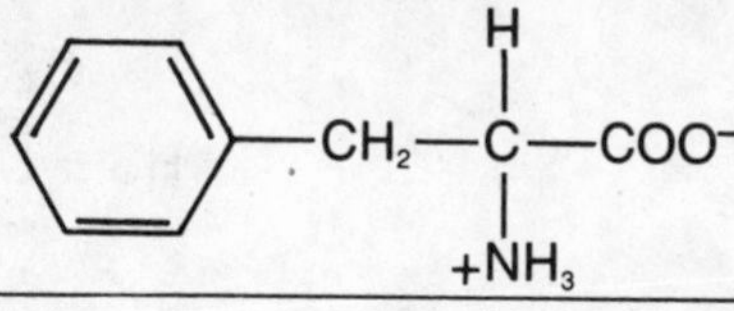

Tryptophan

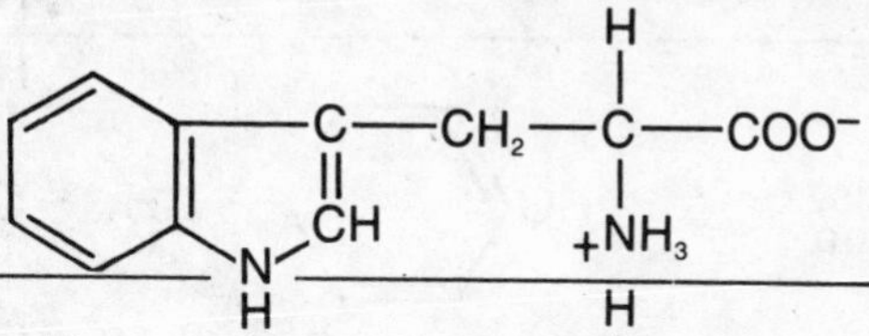

Methionine

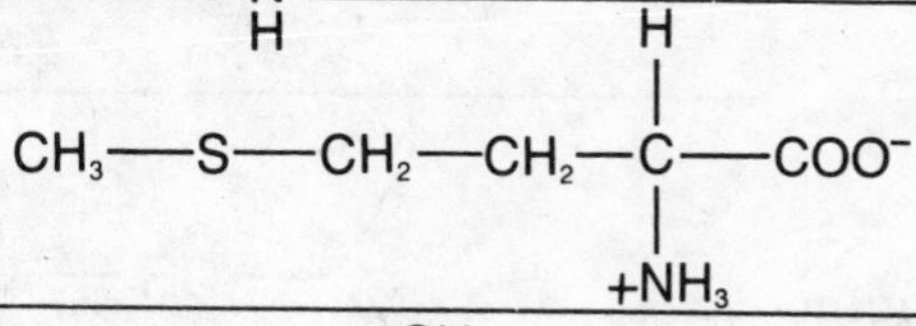

Valine

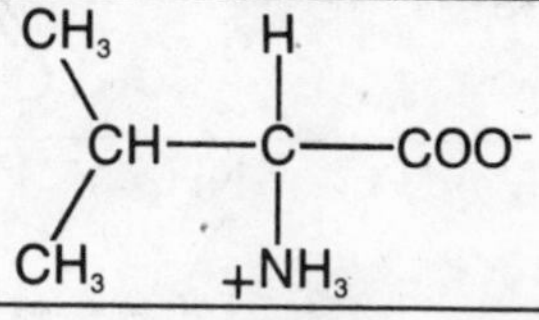

Leucine

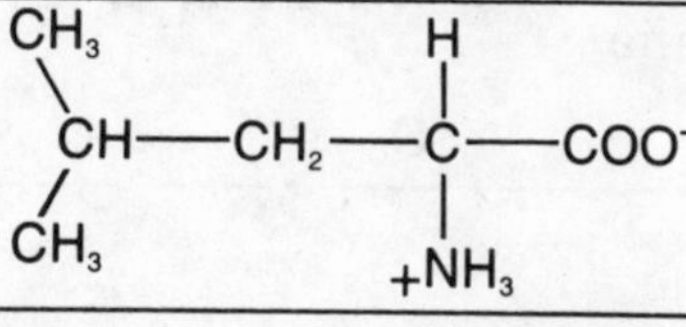

Isoleucine

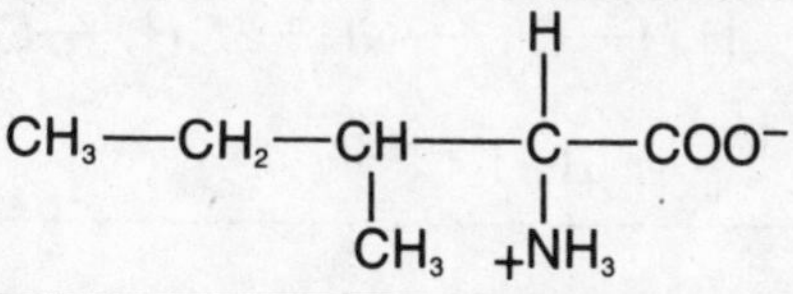

Threonine

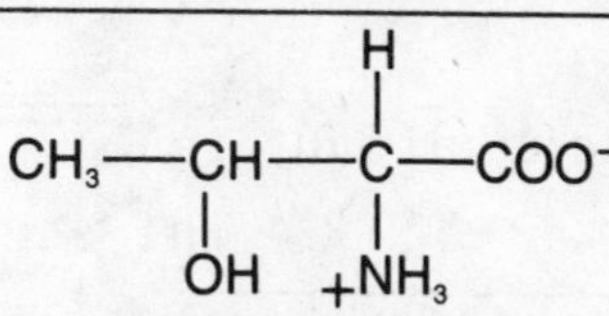

Lysine

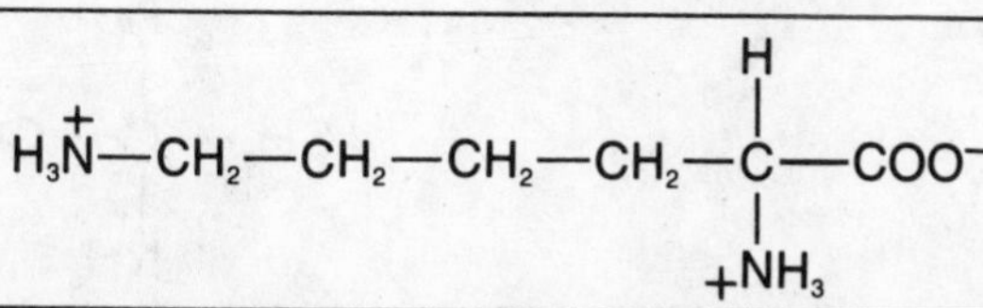

Fourteen Nonessential Amino Acids

Cysteine

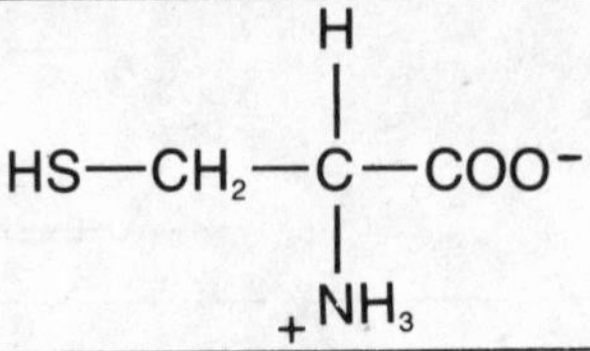

$$HS-CH_2-\underset{\underset{+NH_3}{|}}{\overset{\overset{H}{|}}{C}}-COO^-$$

Tyrosine

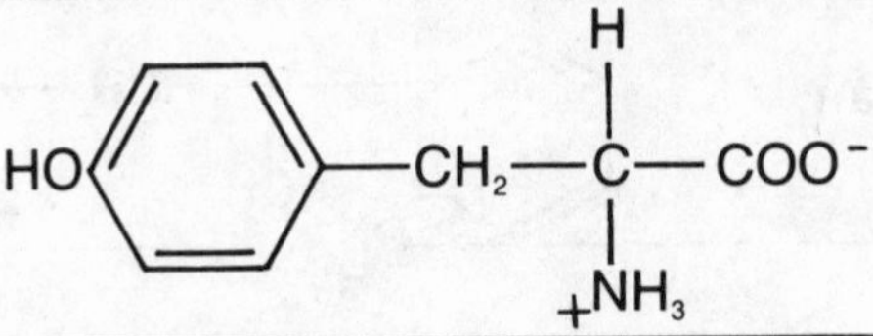

$$HO-\langle\text{ring}\rangle-CH_2-\underset{\underset{+NH_3}{|}}{\overset{\overset{H}{|}}{C}}-COO^-$$

Asparagine

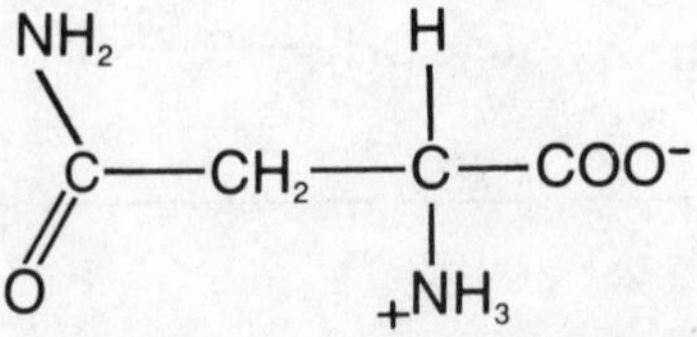

$$\underset{O}{\overset{NH_2}{\underset{\|}{C}}}-CH_2-\underset{\underset{+NH_3}{|}}{\overset{\overset{H}{|}}{C}}-COO^-$$

Glutamine

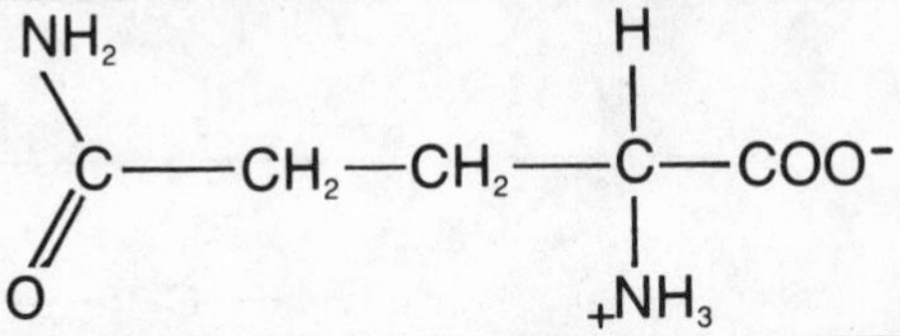

$$\underset{O}{\overset{NH_2}{\underset{\|}{C}}}-CH_2-CH_2-\underset{\underset{+NH_3}{|}}{\overset{\overset{H}{|}}{C}}-COO^-$$

Arginine

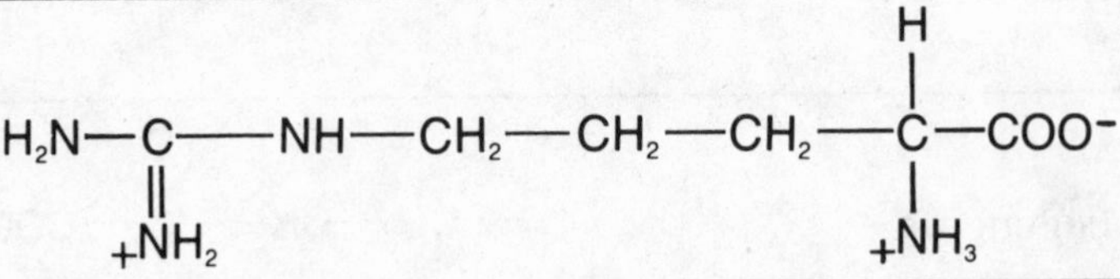

$$H_2N-\underset{\underset{+NH_2}{\|}}{C}-NH-CH_2-CH_2-CH_2-\underset{\underset{+NH_3}{|}}{\overset{\overset{H}{|}}{C}}-COO^-$$

Histidine (at pH 6.0)

$$\underset{\underset{+}{HN}\quad NH}{\overset{HC=C}{\underset{\underset{H}{C}}{}}}-CH_2-\underset{\underset{+NH_3}{|}}{\overset{\overset{H}{|}}{C}}-COO^-$$

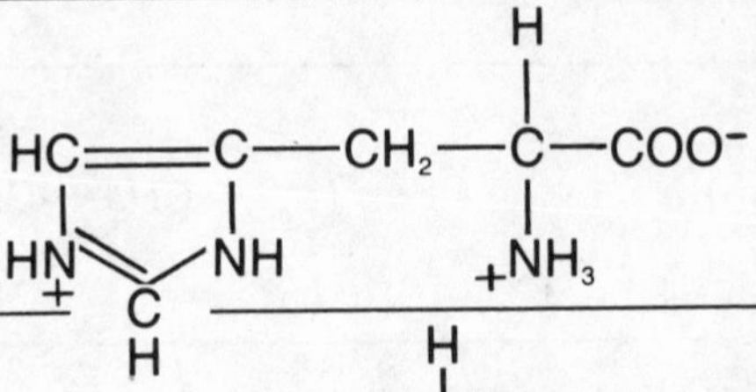

Alanine

$$CH_3-\underset{\underset{+NH_3}{|}}{\overset{\overset{H}{|}}{C}}-COO^-$$

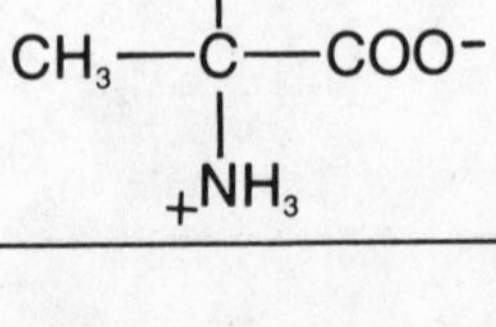

Fourteen Nonessential Amino Acids

Glycine

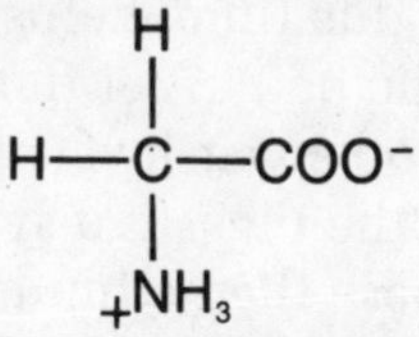

$$H-\underset{\underset{+NH_3}{|}}{\overset{\overset{H}{|}}{C}}-COO^-$$

Serine

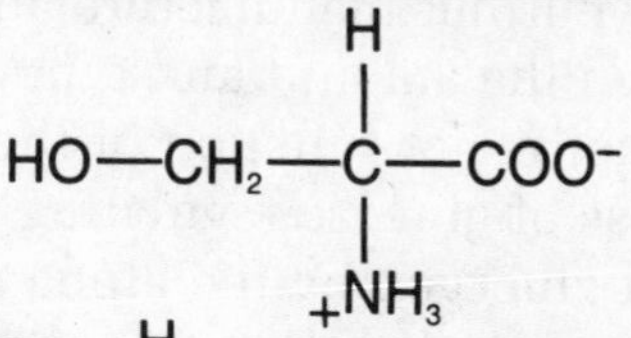

$$HO-CH_2-\underset{\underset{+NH_3}{|}}{\overset{\overset{H}{|}}{C}}-COO^-$$

Proline

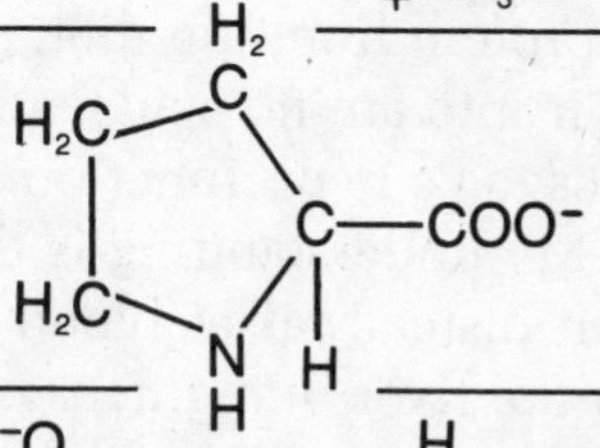

Aspartic acid

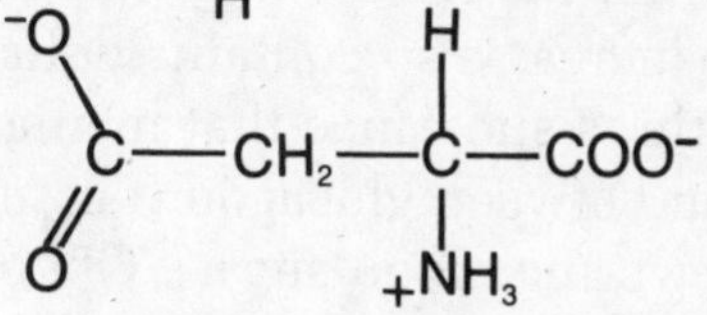

$$\underset{O}{\overset{-O}{\overset{\|}{C}}}-CH_2-\underset{\underset{+NH_3}{|}}{\overset{\overset{H}{|}}{C}}-COO^-$$

Glutamic acid

$$\underset{O}{\overset{-O}{\overset{\|}{C}}}-CH_2-CH_2-\underset{\underset{+NH_3}{|}}{\overset{\overset{H}{|}}{C}}-COO^-$$

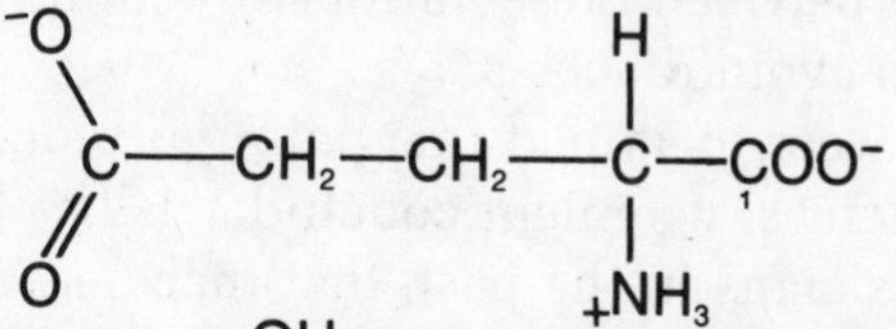

4-hydroxyproline

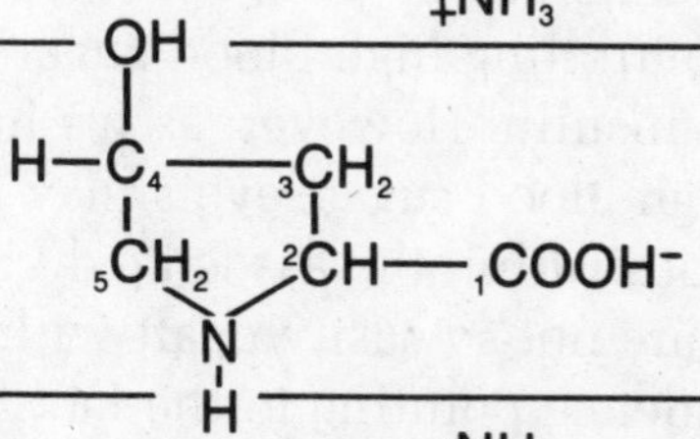

5-hydroxylysine

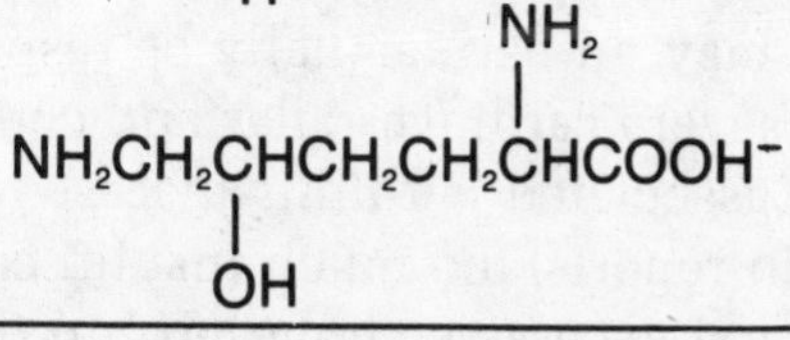

$$NH_2CH_2\underset{\underset{OH}{|}}{CH}CH_2CH_2CHCOOH^-$$

sugar levels within the body; it also simultaneously stimulates the release of insulin. The pancreas, by producing insulin at this time, helps to regulate the level of blood sugar in the body. Yet the production of insulin begins even before blood sugar levels become elevated. As the food we eat enters the digestive system, certain hormones are secreted, and these then stimulate the release of insulin from the beta cells. Further manufacture and release of insulin depends upon the amount and type of food that is eaten.

Another major function of the pancreas contained in this process of glucose regulating metabolism is the production of glucagon by the alpha cells of the gland. The absorption of protein from the diet, and the simultaneous breakdown of it into amino acids, stimulates the release of glucagon. Glucagon's main function is to raise the blood glucose level. My understanding is that glucagon is not anti-insulin but instead raises blood sugar by changing glycogen from the liver *into glucose*.

The pancreas also contains delta cells, which secrete somatostatin, a substance that mediates as a balancing mechanism between glucagon (raising blood sugar) and insulin (lowering blood sugar). Obviously, a proper harmony must exist between these various functions of the pancreas in order to avoid diabetes.

If we were to stop at this point with our examination of the pancreas, we might conclude, as has been done by many physicians in the past, that diabetes is a simple matter of controlling high blood sugar levels by the daily injection of insulin. However, as we have already seen, although high blood sugar levels may indeed be controlled by the use of insulin, the associated killing complications of diabetes are not so easily dealt with. There is, in fact, medical evidence pointing to the fact that daily injections of insulin may, in part, actually be responsible for some of the many severe cardiovascular and cerebrovascular complications associated with this disease. As Dr. Bernard E. Lowenstein reports, too much insulin can stimulate the production of excessive cholesterol in the body.

The insulin made in the body goes from the pancreas via the bloodstream to the liver first where at least half of it is used. Only a small amount then courses through the rest of the body. The rest of the body needs only a small amount. But what happens when you inject insulin under your skin, in your arm or leg or buttocks? It does not go to the liver first, obviously. It goes through the whole peripheral circulation first, then reaches the liver. The result of this is that the whole peripheral circulatory system contains considerably more insulin than it needs. This peripheral hyperinsulinism is a direct result of an insulin injection. The insulin-requiring diabetic must inject enough insulin to meet the needs of the liver, otherwise ketoacidosis will develop. But enough insulin for the liver means too much for the rest of the body. Now you can see why hyperinsulinism is almost unavoidable in insulin-requiring diabetics taking injections. Moreover, we believe it is this hyperinsulinism that contributes to much more severe complications associated with this type of diabetes.

Why should insulin, a natural substance, not an artificial drug, cause these complications? One possibility is that insulin, in more than needed amounts, actually produces fat. One researcher, Dr. R. W. Stout of Hammersmith Hospital in London, actually showed that when laboratory rats were given insulin intravenously, the insulin stimulated the synthesis of cholesterol in the blood vessel wall. Other investigators have shown that when too much insulin is present in the blood, all kinds of "metabolic debris" can be found, including certain chemicals that are found deposited on the insides of blood vessels that have been partly occluded, as in arteriosclerosis.[2]

Since it is true that unavoidably high insulin dosages can seriously aggravate the tiny blood vessel disease so characteristic of diabetes, we must turn our attention to other, alternative approaches that not only control the high blood sugar levels of diabetes but also reduce or eliminate this disease's associated complications. In order to accomplish this, let us continue our examination of the pancreas. For while the endocrine (ductless) function of insulin secretion is well known by many, this gland's all-important exocrine (duct) secretions are relatively unknown by the general public, and their possible connection with a partial cure for diabetes—along with diet and other associated therapies—is still not common knowledge among physicians.

Medical practitioners since the 1920s have been reporting individual maladaptive reactions to foods and chemicals observed as emerging during controlled systematic test exposures. These reactions are especially acute after a four to seven day period of avoidance of incriminating substances. They have been varyingly characterized as allergic, hypersensitive and maladaptive, or enzymatic deficiency reactions. Substances evoking these reactions are far more numerous than the proteins conventionally associated with allergic reactions, and in fact include all food categories and chemicals, especially those most frequently contacted. The types of reactions evoked are as varied as the many tissues and organ systems of the human body; therefore, mental as well as physical symptoms can occur.

The pancreas is the first organ to be influenced by contact with ingested foods and/or chemicals. It has the important task of making useful all metabolic products from the ingested substances and also of protecting the body from reactions to any of these substances. An overstimulated pancreas follows, as we have seen, the same general law that other overstimulated tissues and organ systems follow; overstimulation eventually leads to inhibition of function. All addictions, of course, whether they are to foods of any kind, chemicals, tobacco and/or alcohol, eventually lead to pancreatic insufficiency of varying degrees. But what is important to realize here is that most affected in pancreatic insufficiency of these types are the bicarbonate and enzyme productions of the organ, both of which are exocrine (duct) secretions, and least of all its insulin production or endocrine (ductless) secretion.

To truly appreciate the significance of pancreatic insufficiency, therefore, we need to first examine the basic physiology of the exocrine function of the pancreas. So far in our discussion we have examined the gland's endocrine function, namely, the ductless secretions of hormones, i.e., proinsulin and insulin, and so on. But aside from the manufacture, storage and release of insulin, the pancreas

also has other important functions. The exocrine secretion—
i.e., through ducts—of digestive enzymes and bicarbonate
is a very important aspect of the gland's total function, and
as we shall see later, is often more inhibited during
pancreatic insufficiency than is its insulin production.

One of the essential exocrine functions of the pancreas
is to supply proteolytic enzymes that aid in the digestion of
proteins to amino acids. In this respect, the pancreas has a
very vital role in the digestion of foods. When proteins are
eaten, for example, the pancreas begins to secrete and
release through a duct into the intestines certain enzymes,
i.e., trypsin, chymotrypsin, and carboxypeptidase, that
digest protein foods into simpler substances called amino
acids; these amino acids are then absorbed directly into
the bloodstream and transported throughout the body for
direct use and/or storage. Obviously, the consequence of
an insufficiency of pancreatic proteolytic enzymes is the
poor digestion of proteins to amino acids. With a developing deficiency of amino acids, a chain reaction throughout
the body begins to occur. First of all, proteolytic enzymes
are built from amino acids; if amino acids are deficient, then
these digestive enzymes will also begin to be deficient. By
the same token, if amino acids are deficient, they will fail to
activate the duodenal and jujenal mucosa to produce
cholecystokinin-pancrezyme which in turn evokes proteolytic
enzyme secretions from the pancreas. All this is why a
deficiency in proteolytic enzymes is a double-edged sword:
it leads first to an insufficiency of amino acids, and this in
turn causes a greater deficiency in proteolytic enzymes.

On the other hand, with an amino acid deficiency,
there is more than just a reduced enzyme production from
the pancreas. As we have seen, insulin is composed of
fifty-one amino acids. When these all-important building
blocks of hormones are in short supply, then the quality
and the quantity of insulin production actually begin to
diminish. This, of course, can lead to a deficiency of
insulin with the resulting effect of high blood sugar or
diabetes. Needless to say, any amino acid deficiency is a
very serious problem since the central nervous system,

hormones, organs as well as all other biochemical systems within the human body begin to function improperly when there is a short supply of these necessary nutrients—the very building blocks of life.

Another problem related to pancreatic insufficiency is the gland's lowered lipase activity. Lipase is that enzyme produced by the pancreas that is needed for proper lipid or fat metabolism. Diabetics have been observed to have a characteristically higher than normal level of free fatty acids (lipids) in the blood. Reduced lipase digestive activity of breaking down fats indeed causes the phospholipid-cholesterol ratio in the blood to rise, and this, of course, is the foundation on which arteriosclerosis and other cardio-vascular diseases are built. There will be more on this later, but for now, it is important to see that the pancreatic digestive functions are radically altered when the gland's activities are inhibited, and this can result in very danger-ous biochemical reactions and deficiencies.

Besides the reduced amino acid level in the body, there are other very serious problems associated with the reduced proteolytic (protein digesting) enzyme production; what we have in mind here is the fact that since proteins are not being properly broken down into amino acids, poorly digested and undigested protein particles begin to be absorbed into the bloodstream through the intestinal mu-cosa membranes; poorly digested whole protein particles in the blood, in turn, evoke kinin inflammatory reactions throughout the body. Disturbed metabolic processes like this have some very serious implications: when unusable inflammatory-evoking protein molecules are first absorbed through the intestinal mucosa and circulate in the blood, they reach tissues in partially digested form. As partially digested protein molecules (peptides), they are treated as invaders in the body, and establish kinin mediated inflam-mation (edema) in specific organ or tissue targets. Inflam-mation, of course, eventually leads to injury. Kinin inflammation reactions in the brain alone have been clinically observed to fall into the classic psychiatric degen-

erative diagnostic categories of schizophrenia, manic depression, psychotic depression, hyperkinesis, autism,
hallucinations, delusions and a host of others.[3] In relating
this type of inflammation to diabetes, we must first understand that it can affect any artery wall within the body.
Artery walls have three major layers (going from inside to
outside): the intima, the media, and the adventitia. Lining
the intima is a single layer of endothelial cells. These keep
the red blood cells that flow through the artery from
leaking through the arterial wall, and they also control the
flow of water and other blood constituents into the tissues
in which the artery is imbedded. The intima itself may
contain some cells or just fibrous noncellular material.
And it is here in the intima that arteriosclerosis is thought
to have its greatest effect:

*Any strokes, which occur in the brain, result from a reduced
blood flow in arteries in the head sufficient to cause impaired
brain function and, often, death. Like strokes, heart attacks also
result from a reduced flow of blood in the three arteries
surrounding the heart—the coronary arteries.*

*A reduced flow can be caused by a number of diseases that
affect the blood vessels but the most prevalent—especially in
diabetes—is the disease known as arteriosclerosis, commonly
called "hardening of the arteries." The word arteriosclerosis is
derived from the Greek word "athera," which means gruel—a
soft, pasty material. "Sclerosis" means hardening which is characteristic of the later stages of the disease when calcium and other
materials become deposited on the arterial walls. Arteriosclerosis
can occur in any of our large arteries but it is most commonly
found in the coronary arteries that supply blood to the heart, and
the head and neck arteries that supply blood to the brain. In our
society, the buildup of fatty material in these arteries begins at a
very early age. Blood flow is then reduced by the growing mass
of fatty material in these arteries or by the formation of a blood
clot. Whatever the cause, the flow of blood to some vital organ
(ischemia) is reduced. If that organ is the heart, a heart attack
may occur. When the blood supply to the brain is reduced, a
stroke can result. An appropriate analogy would be the buildup of
rust in an iron pipe over a period of years such that the flow of
water to a vital point like the kitchen sink or the bathtub would*

*be slowed or stopped. Research into the cause of arteriosclerosis
has focused mainly on the lumpy thickening of the arterial wall
called a "plaque."*[4]

As this commentary states, arteriosclerosis is most
common in diabetes. Similarly kinin mediated inflammation, caused by a lack of proteolytic enzyme activity, is also
common in diabetes. But what is the connection between
these two seemingly unrelated events? The answer to this
question comes to us through the fact that kinin mediated
inflammation can, and in many cases does, cause severe
irritation to the intima of the arteries. These damaged
inflamed areas of the arteries are then open to absorb more
circulating lipids (already in greater abundance due to the
reduced lipase enzyme activity of the pancreas) than is
healthy for them to do. The absorption of greater than
normal levels of circulating lipids will eventually cause the
formation of the arteriosclerotic plaque, which is simply a
lump elevated above the normal surface of the inside lining
(intima) of the arterial wall. A plaque can close down or
occlude an artery, but more frequently it provokes the
formation of a blood clot (thrombosis) which, in itself, can
also occlude an artery. Obviously, there are other reasons
than kinin mediated inflammation in the artery wall that
cause the formation of arterial plaques. These conditions,
to be discussed in subsequent chapters, can often be
associated with specific nutrient deficiencies. But what is
important to our discussion now is for all of us to realize
that kinin mediated inflammatory plaque formation, which
can lead to arteriosclerosis, is one degenerative indication
usually associated with diabetes, and is in fact partially a
result of the pancreas's associated exocrine secretion of
proteolytic and lipase enzymes.

Parenthetically speaking, cooking foods above 118
degrees Fahrenheit destroys digestive enzymes. When this
happens, the pancreas, salivary glands, stomach and intestines must all come to the rescue and furnish digestive
enzymes (protease for the proteins, lipase for the fats and
amylase for the carbohydrates) to break down all these

substances. To do this repeatedly, the body must rob, so to speak, enzymes from the other glands, muscles, nerves and the blood to help in its demanding digestive process. Eventually, the glands—and this includes the pancreas—develop deficiencies of enzymes because they have been forced to work harder due to the low level of enzymes found in cooked food. Thus, not only are pancreatic exocrine deficiencies caused by addictive and other maladaptive reactions to foods and/or chemicals, but they can also be related to the stress producing factor of always eating cooked foods in which the naturally occurring digestive enzymes contained in the food are destroyed in the heating process. Clinical evidence that supports this thinking is offered to us by a recent study done at the University of Minnesota by Professor Jackson of the Department of Anatomy. He has shown that rats fed for 155 days on an 80 percent cooked food diet manifested an increased pancreatic weight of 20 to 30 percent with a corresponding decrease of digestive enzyme secretions. And what is true for animals is also true for man. Accordingly, while we know that our body can manufacture enzymes, and in particular pancreatic digestive enzymes, we must also always keep in mind that the more we use our enzyme potential, the faster it is going to run out. When you eat food that is raw, the enzymes contained in the food immediately start breaking down the food that is ingested. Your chances, therefore, of not putting a burden on your pancreas are better if you eat as much raw food as possible.

When too much dietary stress causes the pancreas to function improperly, there is another deficiency that develops in its exocrine function. Related to a diminution of proteolytic enzymes, there is also a reduction in the proper levels of pancreatic bicarbonate. Bicarbonate is that pancreatic secretion which creates a necessary alkaline medium for the small intestines.

The Heidelberg gastro-intestinal analysis examination (Figure 3.2) should be given to all diabetic patients, since

---

HEIDELBERG pH GASTROGRAM

Name _____ Date _____ Fasting _____ Hours _____

Age _____ Sex _____ Weight _____ History of Gastric Surgery? _____

○ ○

ESOPHAGUS

Graph shows typical pH changes during passage of the Heidelberg pH Capsule through the gastrointestinal tract.

8
7
6
5
pH 4
3 STOMACH
2
1

8
6 SMALL INTESTINE
5
pH 4
2 PASSING INTO THE DUODENUM
1

○ ○

Changed pH Solutions _____ Began Test at _____ A.M./P.M. Chart: Slow 72mm/hr. Fast 360mm/hr.

DIAGNOSIS (Check one)

☐ Normal Limits   ☐ Borderline Hypochlorhydria
☐ Hypochlorhydria   ☐ Borderline Hyperchlorhydria
☐ Hyperchlorhydria
☐ Other Observations _____

Stomach pH: _____ Stomach emptied at: _____ A.M./P.M.

Small intestine pH: _____ Completed test at: _____ A.M./P.M.

PHARMACEUTICAL GASTRIC pH CORRECTIVE ACTION
CAUTION! Do not rush test — Allow time for pH adjustment

Pharmaceutical Agent Administered and Dosage

1. _____ at _____ A.M./P.M. pH Results _____ at _____ A.M./P.M.
2. _____ at _____ A.M./P.M. pH Results _____ at _____ A.M./P.M.
3. _____ at _____ A.M./P.M. pH Results _____ at _____ A.M./P.M.
4. _____ at _____ A.M./P.M. pH Results _____ at _____ A.M./P.M.

Interrupted test at: _____ Reason: _____
                                        (e.g.: Acid challenge or delayed emptying)

Carefully mark above corresponding number on graph above the point where you administered pharmaceutical product.

Observation and Remarks: _____
_____

Rx _____
_____

Follow-up test needed: _____ If yes, please return on _____
                        (Yes or No)

HEIDELBERG pH CAPSULE SYSTEM
Electro-Medical Devices, Inc. — Scientific Instruments Division
Atlanta, Georgia 30360

it reveals the presence or absence of normal acid in the stomach as well as the proper bicarbonate production from the pancreas.

Stomach gastric digestion occurs in an acid medium (pH of 1.8 to 3, with best function occurring at a pH of 1.8 to 2), while the small intestine functions in an alkaline medium of pH 6.8 and higher, and best at a pH of 8 to 9. One can see by examining Figure 3.2 that as the Heidelberg pH capsule (or in reality food) passes through the stomach into the small intestine, the pancreas should begin to secrete its bicarbonate production. The secretion raises the small intestine pH level (i.e., 6.8 to 9). In pancreatic deficiencies, acute metabolic acidosis after the meal usually occurs since the pancreatic bicarbonate now undersupplied has not neutralized the acid from the stomach as it empties into the duodenum plus the small intestine. This reduction of proper bicarbonate levels in the pancreas results in a chain reaction whereby the pancreatic proteolytic enzymes, which are also secreted into the small intestine, and which need an alkaline medium in which to function best, are destroyed. Pancreatic proteolytic enzyme deficiency, as we now know, has very serious consequences: 1. there develops a corresponding amino acid deficiency caused by an improper digestion of proteins to amino acids; 2. poorly digested and undigested proteins are absorbed into the blood through the intestinal mucous membrane and evoke kinin and prostaglandin inflammatory reactions throughout the body; 3. and there is a continual rise in kinin and prostaglandin inflammatory reactions in arteries, capillaries, and other tissues and organ targets.

In summary the pancreas is the first endocrine-exocrine organ to be influenced by the ecologic contact with ingested foods and chemicals. In view of such a fact, we can well understand the predisposition of the pancreas as the primary shock organ to ingested foods and chemicals. An overstimulated pancreas follows the same general law that other overstimulated tissues and organ systems follow, namely, that overstimulation eventually leads to inhibition of function. Most affected in pancreatic insufficiency is the bicarbonate and enzyme production (exocrine functions) and least of all insulin production (endocrine function). Chronic addictive reactions and their counterpart reactions to foods, chemicals and inhalants are the central stress factors, along with—as we shall see—nutrient deficiencies in diet, that produce the pancreatic deficiency disease process. Once the pancreas begins to function poorly, we encounter an acute metabolic acidosis occurring in the small intestines. This reduction of pancreatic bicarbonate destroys proteolytic enzymes; a lower proteolytic enzyme level in the small intestine in turn creates amino acid deficiencies while the correspondingly low proteolytic enzyme level in the blood allows a continual rise in kinin and prostaglandin inflammatory reactions to occur in various tissues and organs. In addition, pancreatic insufficiency is responsible for a lowered lipase activity and higher lipid levels in the blood. The degenerative disease process now begins, and if it continues for any protracted period, these multiple deficiencies feed upon each other and add to the additional metabolic stress that finally breaks up the entire biochemical balance needed for health.

But now the obvious question arises: granted that there can be deficiencies in the pancreas's exocrine function of secreting proteolytic enzymes and bicarbonate, and that deficiencies in amino acids can be established because of this exocrine malfunction, what has all this to do with insulin and diabetes? The answer to this important question will give us the proper foundation upon which to build a solid understanding of the diabetic disease process.

Deficiencies in the exocrine function of the pancreas have been scientifically observed to be associated with pancreatic endocrine insulin deficiencies as far back as 1925. Abnormal exocrine-pancreatic function has been reported in patients with juvenile-onset and maturity-onset diabetes by many investigators.[5] The most recent study discussing the relationships between endocrine and exocrine deficiencies in the pancreas is offered to us by Dr. B. M. Frier. The results of this study are as follows:

Exocrine pancreatic function was studied in twenty juvenile-onset diabetics, seven maturity-onset diabetics, and five patients with diabetes secondary to chronic pancreatitis. The outputs of bicarbonate and proteolytic enzymes of all the groups of diabetic patients were significantly reduced compared with nondiabetic patients. . . . In the present study exocrine pancreatic secretory capacity was found to be reduced, compared with normal subjects, in 80 percent of insulin-dependent diabetics, and the degree of dysfunction increased with the duration of the disease. . . . Overall, 80 percent of the insulin-dependent patients had abnormal outputs of proteolytic enzymes. . . . All except one of the patients with diabetes of more than five years' duration had an abnormal bicarbonate-secretory response. The incidences of low bicarbonate-secretory capacities therefore are much more common and severe than previously reported. Although the precise cause has not yet been defined, we conclude that exocrine pancreatic dysfunction in insulin-dependent diabetics is a real and significant feature of the disease, and must be taken into account when attempting assessment of exocrine pancreatic function in patients who have diabetes.[6]

The significance of the preceding study offers convincing evidence that diabetes mellitus must encompass a generalized concept of pancreatic insufficiency involving the gland's endocrine as well as exocrine functions. Although Dr. Frier states that "the cause of the exocrine-endocrine deficiency in the pancreas has not yet been defined," we believe, based on clinical findings, that the stress factors of maladaptive allergic-like addictive [likely non-immunologic] responses to incriminating foods and chemicals are its major sources.

Once pancreatic exocrine function is inhibited in diabetes mellitus, and the stress of addictive responses continues, the gland's endocrine function also begins to be inhibited. However, since these addictive responses to foods and chemicals do indeed lead to the pancreatic exocrine dysfunction first, with the resulting amino acid deficiency as discussed earlier, we further believe that, since insulin is composed entirely of amino acids, we must first supplement the diabetic with the exocrine factors of bicarbonate and proteolytic enzymes, as well as amino acids, while simultaneously eliminating the maladaptive reactive foods and chemicals that are inhibiting the pancreatic exocrine function in the first place. Why do this, you ask? Because the enzymes need an alkaline base (bicarbonate) in which to function best. Proteolytic enzymes are needed in order to completely break down proteins into amino acids. And amino acids are essential as the building blocks not only for insulin but for all the cells of the pancreas as well as other glands, organs and life systems within the body.

If such a program is followed, diabetes becomes a reversible abnormal metabolic state in which the stress factors that are inhibiting the proper function of the pancreas are removed, and supportive supplementation for the gland's weakened secretory functions are simultaneously administered. We thus seek the normalization of insulin production by first avoiding addictive substances and next by supplementing pancreatic exocrine function as has already been observed by Dr. David Graham. Dr. Graham discovered, while supplementing pancreatic exocrine insufficiency, other factors such as a positive nitrogen balance, a return of a sense of well-being, and a stabilization and/or a reduction in insulin requirements were often accomplished.[7]

It may seem bold to state but, as our clinical cases will demonstrate, the majority of our maturity-onset type diabetics who follow the preceding program as outlined do not need insulin injections. It has become evident, however, that they do need the exocrine pancreatic supplementation of enzymes, bicarbonate and amino acids. With this type of supplementation, coupled with a reduction in maladaptive substances, we can actually reduce the need for insulin injections.

Case Histories: Exocrine Influence on the Endocrine Function of the Pancreas

This example is taken from the case of a fifty-year-old diabetic. With no supplements given, the food beef originally evoked a blood sugar level of 240 mg percent (diabetes) after one hour post test meal. A test was done to discover the value of exocrine pancreatic supplementation in her case. Thirty minutes before the second test meal, 1260 mg of pancreas compound plus 15 grams of amino acids were given. The 1260 mg of pancreas compound, of course, contained high levels of proteolytic enzymes. With the test meal of beef there was administered 1260 mg of pancreas compound plus 15 grams of free amino acids. The blood sugar before the test was 90 mg percent. Fifteen minutes after the conclusion of the test meal, we again administered 1260 mg of pancreas compound and 15 grams of free amino acids plus 10 grams of sodium bicarbonate. One hour after the test meal her blood sugar was only 140 mg percent (normal). This was a drop of 100 mg percent.

The normalization of pancreatic endocrine function by supplementing pancreatic exocrine function has been observed in our clinic hundreds of times. As more and more case histories revealed this same evidence, it became clear to us that diabetics often need pancreatic exocrine supplementation more than pancreatic endocrine (insulin) support. The schedule of exocrine supplementation can be as follows:

1. At thirty minutes before a meal, a protease supplement is provided. This is supplied from different types of proteases which are not acid labile and therefore are not destroyed by the stomach's gastric acidity. They include: bromelain, papain, liquid aloe vera, liquid aged garlic (kyolic), honey that has not been heated, and superoxide dismutase. These should be selected on a rotation basis (see Chapter 4). Bromelain comes from pineapple and is supplied as 100–500 mg. Papain is usually associated with the bromelain, or bromelain can be obtained separately. Liquid aloe vera is loaded with proteases of various types, and the dose ranges from one to three teaspoons. Kyolic is provided as one capsule of liquid. Unheated (organic) honey ranges from one to three teaspoons. These various proteases exert a normalizing control over maladaptive responses to food and chemicals, and therefore are also used to control blood sugar levels in the body.

2. At the beginning of the meal, glutamic acid hydrochloride and/or butane hydrochloride, or a digestive enzyme tablet containing these, plus pepsin, can be provided in the event there has been a demonstrated clinical deficiency of acid in the stomach. This situation does not occur very frequently.

3. At the end of the meal, give one to two pancreas substance capsules or tablets. These can be obtained from sources of either lamb, beef, pork or aspergillus, and can be rotated on the specific days these food items are used. The end of the meal is the most appropriate time to give any amino acid supplements. These supplements should be given on a specific basis according to the laboratory findings for each individual. Since these are free amino acids, they do not need to be digested, and therefore can be taken at the end of the meal. Sometimes they are given thirty minutes before the meal as a buffer against maladaptive reactions. If a patient should require a suppression of appetite, it would be well to take tyrosine. Five hundred to a thousand milligrams thirty minutes before a meal will offer a sense of satisfaction to the individual and will thus cut down his appetite for food. If this sense of satisfaction is not needed, then tyrosine (an amino acid) should be given on an individual need basis after meals.

4. Thirty to forty-five minutes after the meal, give one of the pancreas substance capsules or tablets again. The number given will range from one to five depending on the person's actual need for better digestion. At this time, an alkalinization is also provided. This usually consists of 10 grains of sodium and potassium bicarbonate. Alternatives to this particular ratio are the same amounts of sodium bicarbonate, calcium bicarbonate, and potassium bicarbonate. These various ratios can be used to supply specific nutrients that have been demonstrated as deficient by laboratory assay. It is also possible at this time to use ascorbates as a neutralizing agent. These can be taken as sodium ascorbate, potassium ascorbate, calcium ascorbate, or magnesium ascorbate. The patient can maintain this program for two to four months and then reduce doses according to individual needs. The chosen source of bicarbonate is given to produce the alkali base needed for activation of the pancreatic enzymes. It should be given thirty to forty-five minutes after the meal, because this is when more solid particles of digestion are being emptied. If there is any gastric distress earlier than this time, the alkali could

be given sooner. Bear in mind that the goal of this treatment is to have the local intestinal alkali high enough to provide an alkali media for the proper function of proteolytic digestive enzymes. It also provides proper absorption of proteolytic enzymes as well as a systemic postmeal activation of the proteolytic enzyme pool or residual supply of proteolytic enzymes in the blood. Such an enzyme pool, in turn, prevents kinin and prostaglandin mediated inflammatory reactions from occurring in response to undigested protein molecules.

More case histories

The following case histories clearly demonstrate the fact that when the exocrine function of the pancreas is supplemented with proteolytic enzymes, bicarbonate and amino acids, maladaptive hyperglycemic reactions to specific foods and chemicals can be controlled. The result of this is that the gland's endocrine function of insulin secretion is normalized. The first patient that witnesses to this fact is Kathy B. After a four day fast, Kathy was observed to react to fourteen foods, of which nine evoked severe high blood sugar reactions. Milk—a protein and fat food—was one of these nine. Before the test meal with milk, her fasting blood sugar was 80 mg percent. After this, she was given milk and her blood sugar was immediately evaluated to 200 mg percent at one hour after the test meal. There were symptoms of nervousness, marked tension, trembling and anger in response to this milk test meal. Four days later we decided to run another milk test meal on Kathy. But this time, in addition to the milk test meal, we would supplement with proteolytic enzymes, bicarbonate and amino acids. At the beginning of the test, her fasting blood sugar was again observed to be 80 mg percent. She was symptom-free. At this time she was given 1670 mg pancreatic enzymes and 15 grams of amino acids. Thirty minutes after this Kathy was symptom-free. The milk test meal was then given. Forty-five minutes after the test meal, her blood sugar was still 80 mg percent. She was also symptom-free. A quarter teaspoon of sodium bicarbonate was then given. One hour later her blood sugar was measured at 90 mg percent, and she was still symptom-free. The results of these two tests clearly indicate that the milk test meal without proteolytic enzymes, bicarbonate and amino acids produced severe hyperglycemia and marked symptoms. However, the milk test meal with these three ingredients produced no symptoms and blood sugar remained normal.

Another interesting case history is Ken J. After a four day fast, Ken was observed to react to twenty-three different foods of which fourteen evoked severe high blood sugar reactions. Pineapple was one of these foods that caused the diabetic reaction. After the fast, Ken's blood sugar was 80 mg percent. The test meal of pineapple was then given and his blood sugar soared to 260 mg percent. The normal post test meal range is between 120 and 160 mg percent. No subjective or objective symptoms, however, were observed. Four days later we again ran a pineapple food test, but this time we supplemented the test with proteolytic enzymes, bicarbonate and amino acids. After a fast and at the beginning of the pineapple food test, Ken was symptom-free and his blood sugar was 80 mg percent. He was given 1,225 mg of concentrated enzymes plus 15 grams of amino acids. Thirty minutes after this his blood sugar was still 80 mg percent and he was symptom-free. The test meal of pineapple was then given. One hour after the test meal his blood sugar was still normal, registering 130 mg percent. He was also symptom-free. At this time he was given a quarter teaspoon of sodium bicarbonate. An hour after this his blood sugar was still 130 mg percent and he was completely symptom-free. The results of this test again indicate that diabetes was present on the pineapple test without any supplementation of proteolytic enzymes, bicarbonate or amino acids. Blood sugar, however, remained normal on the test after supplementation was given.

Another example with more severe hyperglycemic reactions is revealed to us by Mary J., a twenty-seven-year-old diabetic schizophrenic. After a four day fast, Mary's blood sugar was 100 mg percent. A test meal for raisins was given without any form of supplementation. One hour after the test meal with raisins, her blood sugar skyrocketed to 400 mg percent (severe diabetic reaction)! Her symptoms were marked tension, trembling, irritability and unprovoked anger at her mother. Four days later, we decided to test Mary with raisins again; however, this time we would supplement with proteolytic enzymes, amino acids and bicarbonate. She was symptom-free at the beginning of the test. Her blood sugar was 100 mg percent. She was given 1,670 mg of pancreatic enzyme concentrate and 15 grams of amino acids. Thirty minutes after this, the blood sugar was still 100 mg percent. The test meal of raisins was then given. Thirty minutes after the test meal her blood sugar was normal at 160 mg percent. She was also symptom-free. A quarter teaspoon of sodium bicarbonate was administered at this time. One hour after this her blood sugar was 120 mg percent and she was symptom-free. Again, the results of these two tests indicate that without proteolytic enzymes, bicarbonate and amino acids a severe diabetic hyperglycemia with marked symptoms was produced. A test meal with supplementation produced no symptoms and blood sugar remained normal.

Another example illustrating our point was observed with John M., a seventeen-year-old diabetic with multiple food allergies. John had always loved eating chicken, and he ate it almost daily. After a four day fast, we decided to run a chicken food test. A test meal with chicken without any form of supplementation produced a severe depression, poor comprehension, withdrawal, and flat affect. John's blood sugar at one hour post test meal was a startling 300 mg percent. A week later we decided to run another chicken test meal, except this time we would supplement with proteolytic enzymes, bicarbonate and amino acids. John was symptom-free before the test, and his blood sugar was 70 mg percent. At this time we gave him, 1,670 mg of pancreatic concentrated proteolytic enzymes, plus 15 grams of free amino acids. Thirty minutes after step 1 his blood sugar remained at 70 mg percent, and there were no symptoms observed. At this time, John sat down and ate a medium

sized chicken meal. Thirty minutes after this supplemented
test meal, his blood sugar was a normal 100 mg percent, and
no symptoms were observed. We then also gave him a
quarter teaspoon of sodium bicarbonate. One hour later, his
blood sugar was a normal 100 mg percent, and no objective symptoms were observed. John said he felt very well.
As expected in John's case, there was a marked difference
in symptoms and blood sugar levels between the test meal
given with supplementation and the one given without.

Foods are not the only substances that produce severe
diabetic reactions and marked pancreatic deficiencies.
Chemicals also have power to alter pancreatic production of
proteolytic enzymes, bicarbonate, as well as insulin secretions. Back in 1970, a revealing study of the effects of
chronic exposure to air pollution was done by Dr. P. U.
Capurro in a small town near Elkton, Máryland. At that
time, strong odors were detected, particularly at night,
over a two mile area inhabited by approximately one
hundred people. These odors were described as "glue-
like," "disagreeable," "pungent," "vomit-like" or "peppermint-
like." The odors had a tendency to localize in pockets
along the valley of the small town. In the valley, there was a
chemical plant that recovered solvents from discarded
chemical materials. An officer of the company stated to Dr.
Capurro that they distilled alcohol and methylethyl ke-
tone. The state of Maryland informed him that the company
also processed "fusel oil" (which has as its chief constitu-
ent isoamyl alcohol). They also informed him that benzene
was present in some of their materials. Of the forty-three
people that Dr. Capurro observed, all of whom were chronically exposed to these chemical substances, all forty-three
expressed symptoms of fatigue, thirty-three expressed symptoms of irritability, thirty-two had periods of absentmind-
edness, thirty had achy feelings, twenty-eight expressed
sensations of lightheadedness, and thirty-two had chronic
headaches. Other symptoms experienced by the forty-three
people included persistent infections, burning throats,
burning eyes, nausea, chest pains, depression and confusion. After further testing, Dr. Capurro discovered that a

high percentage of these people had abnormal blood sugar curves and concluded that the chemical pollution actually was damaging the endocrine portion of the pancreas. After more testing, Dr. Capurro also discovered that there was exocrine damage to the pancreas. "We have," he writes, "a major manifestation of damage to the pancreas that shows itself on the exocrine portion of the gland . . . and on the endocrine portion of the gland, as demonstrated by elevated fasting blood sugars and/or abnormal glucose tolerance." Dr. Capurro concluded, after all his testing, that "the organ most damaged by the air pollution was the pancreas, followed by the lung and then the liver and the kidney."[8]

Dr. Capurro's conclusions concerning the relationship existing between certain chemical air pollutants and severe diabetic reactions were observed to be valid in our clinical testing of diabetic patients. Frank M., a twenty-three-year-old diabetic, was sublingually (under the tongue) tested with minute amounts of auto exhaust fumes. Before the test, Frank had a blood fasting level of 90 mg percent. After the exposure, there were immediate symptoms of marked negativism, loss of insight, reduced ability to concentrate, reduced comprehension and a painful tension in the back of the neck. His blood sugar soared to a surprising 320 mg percent. We decided to run the same test a week later, but this time we would supplement with proteolytic enzymes, bicarbonate and amino acids. At the beginning of the test, Frank's fasting sugar level was 90 mg percent and there were no objective or subjective symptoms noted. We administered 1,670 mg of pancreatic enzymes concentrate. Thirty minutes after this the sublingual test of auto exhaust fumes was given. Also at this time, 15 grams of free amino acids plus a quarter teaspoon of sodium bicarbonate were given. Thirty minutes after the administration of supplements as well as the sublingual auto exhaust fumes test, there were no major observable symptoms. His blood sugar was a normal 150 mg percent. There was, however, a minor and brief nasal stuffiness at the beginning of the test. What this study reveals to us is that while specific chemical air pollutants can indeed, as Dr. Capurro has proven, create an exocrine-endocrine pancreatic disorder, proper exocrine supplementation coupled with amino acids can strengthen an individual's ability to defend against the altered blood sugar levels induced by a specific allergic (immunologic) allergic-like (non-immunologic enzyme inhibition) or addictive reaction to these chemical pollutants.

Case history: a juvenile diabetic

The juvenile diabetic often has maladaptive reactions to his environment because he does not possess adequate proteolytic enzymes to control kinin and prostaglandin inflammatory reactions. Therefore, even though the juvenile type diabetic will remain insulin dependent, he does very definitely need Bio-Ecologic diagnosis and treatment. A case history of John, age eighteen, who was diabetic most of his life and at the time of examination was receiving sixty units of insulin a day, illustrates this point. His blood pressure was 180/110. There was four plus protein spillage in his urine. He had a general sense of weakness and tension. His eyes had already deteriorated to the extent that he had received laser treatment for both of them. He was first tested for allergies and other maladaptive reactions at our clinic. When the foods, chemicals and inhalants to which he was reactive were removed, and when he was placed on the appropriate levels of bicarbonate and proteolytic enzymes as well as other nutrients, his insulin requirement dropped from the initial sixty units to only twenty units per day. He was found to be symptom reactive to a wide assortment of foods and chemicals. At the time of the completion of his assessment one month later, his blood pressure was 130/80. There was no protein spillage in the urine; he felt strong and was requiring only twenty units of insulin.

This case is an example of what has happened with several other juvenile diabetics when Bio-Ecologic diagnosis and treatment was administered. The evidence strongly suggests that even the juvenile diabetic does not have to physically deteriorate and suffer, a position which until recently was classically accepted as inevitable.

Summary

The previously mentioned studies based on biochemical monitoring of glucose before and during induction test exposures to foods and chemicals reveal that the diabetes mellitus disease process involves a total disordered pancreatic function rather than only a selected disordered insulin production, as previously believed. The most seriously curtailed function is that of reduced production of bicarbonate, followed by reduced proteolytic enzyme production, and finally by reduced insulin production. The pancreas, therefore, is the first endocrine-exocrine organ to be influenced by the ecologic contact with ingested foods and chemicals. As continued contact with specific foods and chemicals creates addictions, the pancreas, due to the demands of this overstimulation and overwork, begins to show signs of inhibition of function. The consequences of insufficient exocrine pancreatic function are: 1. acute metabolic acidosis post meal, since the pancreatic bicarbonate has not properly neutralized the acid from the stomach as it empties into the duodenum; 2. the simultaneous inactivation of and/or destruction of proteolytic enzymes (trypsin, chymotrypsin and carboxypeptidase) from the pancreas; 3. poor digestion of proteins to amino acids; 4. unusable inflammation evoking protein molecules being absorbed through the intestinal mucosa, circulating in the blood, reaching tissues in undigested form, and evoking both immunologic (histamine) as well as nonimmunologic (kinin and prostaglandin) inflammatory reactions in any area of the body, including the brain, heart, arteries. This then destroys the body's ability to make other enzymes, hormones (including insulin), tissues, as well as antibodies against infection, and also creates a very excessive demand not only for vitamins, but for minerals, trace elements and other metabolites used by the body for literally millions of chemical reactions.

Since the stress of addiction is the first and most important factor starting all the preceding chain reactions of the pancreatic degenerative disease process, it would seem wise, as a first step, to attempt to stop the stress of addictive contacts with food and chemicals. On the other hand, it would seem unwise to use only proteolytic enzymes, bicarbonate and amino acid supplementation in the expectation of a miraculous cure of diabetes. Certainly this supplementation program does play an important role in the control of diabetes, and as shown, can even significantly reduce the need for insulin therapy. However, if the continual and central stress factor of addiction is not resolved, this chronic abuse will eventually inhibit the pancreas to such a degree that the exocrine supplements of enzymes and bicarbonate, coupled with amino acids, will begin to be less effective. Therefore, a regime must be established whereby the mechanism of blocking maladaptive reactions to foods and chemicals is controlled. This method of keeping maladaptive food exposures reduced or spaced below the frequency that evokes symptoms is called a diversified rotation diet.

REFERENCES

1. Williams, R. J. and Kalita, D. K. 1979. *A Physician's Handbook on Orthomolecular Medicine.* New Canaan, CT.: Keats Publishing, p. 2.

2. Lowenstein, B.E. 1976. *Diabetes.* New York: Harper and Row, pp. 39–40.

3. Kalita, D. K. and Philpott, W. H. 1980. *Brain Allergies: The Psycho-Nutrient Connection.* New Canaan, CT.: Keats Publishing.

4. *Executive Health* (August 1979) XV:11.

5. Baron, J. H. 1973. Pancreatic exocrine function in maturity-onset diabetes mellitus. *British Medical Journal* 4:25–27; Bock, O. A. 1967. Exocrine pancreatic function in diabetes mellitus. *South African Medical Journal* 41:756–758; Chey, W. Y. 1963.

External pancreatic secretion in diabetes mellitus. *Annals of Internal Medicine* 59:812–821; Diamond, J. S. 1940. The secretin test in the diagnosis of pancreatic disease with a report of 130 tests. *American Journal of Digestive Diseases* 7:435–442; Domschke, W. 1975. Exocrine pancreatic function in juvenile diabetes. *American Journal of Digestive Diseases* 20:309–312; Drewes. V. M. 1969. Exocrine pancreatic function. *Modern Gastroenterology.* eds. Gregor and Riedl, Stuttgart: Schattauer, pp. 1229–1231; Jones, C. M. 1925. Pancreatic and hepatic activity in diabetes mellitus. *Archives of Internal Medicine* 35:315–336; Pollard, H. M. 1943. The external secretion of the pancreas and diabetes mellitus. *American Journal of Digestive Diseases* 10-20-23; Vacca, J. B. 1964. The exocrine pancreas in diabetes mellitus. *Annals of Internal Medicine* 61:837–848; Yamagata, S. 1969. Exocrine and endocrine function of the pancreas in diabetes mellitus. *Modern Gastroenterology,* pp. 1298–1300.

6. Frier, B. M. 1976. Exocrine pancreatic function in juvenile-onset diabetes mellitus. *Gut* 17:685–691.

7. Graham, D. Y. 1977. Enzyme replacement therapy of exocrine pancreatic insufficiency in man. *New England Journal of Medicine* 296:1314–1317.

8. Capurro, P. U. 1970. Effects of chronic exposure to solvents caused by air pollution. *Clinical Toxicology* 2:233–248.

CHAPTER FOUR

The diversified rotation diet

After one has successfully diagnosed food and chemical maladaptive allergic reactions, the next obvious goal is to establish some kind of control whereby these maladaptive reactions—and their associated addictions—can be completely avoided. The most reliable method of obtaining this goal is a diversified rotation diet.

Fanny Lou Leeney, M.D., allergist, was the first to use a diversified rotation diet. Herbert Rinkel, M.D., allergist, while practicing in Oklahoma City, Oklahoma, adopted the diversified rotation diet from Dr. Leeney. Dr. Rinkel, using his understanding of masked food allergy or "food addiction" (Theron G. Randolph, 1956), demonstrated that a symptom producing food does not have to be abandoned forever but can be returned to the diet if this is done after sufficient time for the body to completely recover from the initial maladaptive food reaction. More specifically, in order to stop the vicious cycle of addiction, foods that give minor reactions should be avoided for a minimum of six weeks; then they should be eaten no more often than every four days. Foods that give major reactions should be avoided for a minimum of three months; thereafter they too should be eaten every four days and only once in four days. If reactions occur on this program, incriminating foods should be avoided for another month, and tried again. The principle is to avoid the symptom evoking substance until the refractory phase (i.e., that stage in which the allergic or allergic-like state is broken) of the healing process develops after a few days, weeks, or months. It is important to realize that the refractory phase usually begins at about three weeks, and is well established by three months of complete avoidance. No food addictions are likely to develop once the refractory stage has occurred and a four-day rotation diet is practiced.

In 1971, we started, under the supervision of Marshall Mandell, M.D., allergist, to systematically test patients by deliberate exposure to single foods. We found that a food fast using nonchemically treated water only gave us our best results of improvement as well as evidence of a cause and effect relationship between food addiction and symptom reactions. At that time, Dr. Theron G. Randolph, and Dr. Marshall Mandell, both advised a diversified rotation diet. Initially, this diet seemed so difficult that, for a number of patients, I used a method of allowing free and frequent use of their nonreactive foods (i.e., foods that produced no symptoms). A few months later, I admitted several of these patients back to the hospital. Retesting revealed they were again sick due to the establishment of new addictions to a new set of what were once nonreactive foods and which they now were eating frequently. It proved to be disastrous to allow frequent use of any foods. I therefore sought the most rigid separation of foods to prevent this reinstatement of addiction. In discussing my problem with several experienced ecologists, I adopted the advice of John McLennon, M.D., allergist. He suggested that I keep the foods in families and space their contact four days apart. I asked Ruth Nielson, R.D., dietitian at Fuller Memorial Hospital, where I was doing this work, to arrange diets with foods in families and with one food member per family eaten every four days.

Foods theoretically should be rotated in families every four days since there may be a cross-allergic reaction between family members. For example, lemon, orange, grapefruit, lime, tangerine, kumquat and citron are all of the citrus family. If symptoms are evoked by this family of foods, then each food within the family should be first avoided for three months and then rotated on a four-day basis. More specifically, this means that if I eat an orange on Monday, I should not eat any other member of the family until Friday of that same week. It is important to understand that even though this procedure requires specific dietary planning, and is often, from a practical standpoint, difficult to achieve, it does reduce allergic reactions as well as increase one's exposure to a broader spectrum of nutrients.

But as the years progressed, I became convinced that the theoretical proposition of eating only one member of a food family every four days was a very demanding regime and was not necessary for all my patients. As a result, I adopted what has been called a "maximum restrictive diversified rotation diet"—either on a four or seven day basis for the more severely allergic patient—or a "minimum restrictive four day diversified rotation diet" for those who manifest less severe allergic/addictive responses.

Dr. Theron G. Randolph has had the most years of experience in the area of diet and human ecology, and, therefore, has been most meticulous in his applications and observations about the diversified rotation diet. His "maximum restrictive diversified rotation diet" has become the standard of excellence in the field. His conclusions are that the most efficient program is: 1. single foods, whether initially symptom reactive or not, should be eaten once only in four days; 2. foods are restricted to the same family on the day a food is eaten; 3. one day must intervene between the use of any two members of a family. For example, whereas wheat would not be eaten more frequently than once in four days, another member of this cereal grain family (e.g., oats) could be eaten as a single meal on the third day of the rotation, with wheat again being eaten on the first day of the next cycle, i.e., the fifth day. He also believes that the least number of foods eaten in a single meal reduces the chances of a reaction occurring. Whereas several foods may be successfully eaten by most people, only one, two or three foods at a meal may be necessary for a few severely sensitive reactors. This is very likely based on a selective inability of a given person to provide adequate digestive enzymes and/or other metabolic factors to handle the metabolism of the multiple foods.

Patients should be taught to return to the foods to which they were initially demonstrated to be symptom-reactive. It is important that they not try to follow the total rejection of these foods for the rest of their lives. Often these are foods that are valuable for good nutrition. If they find they cannot reinstate these at three months, they should try at four months or five months. If they find that they cannot rotate them once in four days, they should try once in eight days or once in two weeks or once a month.

A minority of subjects have fixed food reactions. These are usually easy to spot because each time the person eats the food, symptoms develop in spite of avoidance and/or rotation. Certain incriminating chemicals fall into this category. In the case of fixed food or chemical allergy, the substance must be avoided completely at all times. Any type of program such as described above will not help a fixed food reaction; only complete avoidance will stop reactions in these cases.

There is no way other than rotation to assure a non-reactive state to initially symptom incriminative foods. However, there are some degrees of protection provided by adequate nutrition. In examining patients, it is often demonstrated in the laboratory that they are deficient in vitamin C, B6, folic acid, chromium, zinc, magnesium, manganese and so forth. Providing these necessary nutrients, as well as others, is an aid in reducing the maladaptive reactivity to the foods. A detailed examination of all these different Bio-ecologic aspects of treatment will be given in subsequent chapters, but for now, we must always remember that the rotation diet is the first and most important weapon used in the battle against addictions.

Summary of the maximum restrictive diversified four day rotation diet

1. Eat no single food more often than once in four days. This applies whether these foods were initially symptom-evoking or not.

2. Foods are kept in families so that members of a specific family are used only on the days assigned to that family. (See Maximum Restrictive Diversified Four Day Rotation Diet chart.)

3. The use of members of food families is kept two days apart. An exception is that in the case of cereal grains rice and millet can be used two days after cereal grains containing gluten such as wheat, rye, barley and buckwheat.

4. The fewer the number of foods used in a single meal, the less chance of a maladaptive reaction. Some highly reactive people can eat only one, two or three foods at a meal while less reactive people can eat a much larger variety at a single meal.

5. The larger the amount of food eaten the greater the chance of a reaction. Therefore, moderate servings are more optimal than large servings.

Other considerations for the maximum restrictive four day diversified rotation diet

1. For some, allergic reactions will occur if a food is eaten on a single exposure four day rotation basis whereas a reaction may not occur if spaced on a single exposure eight day, sixteen day, or thirty-two day basis.

2. Any time a food is suspected as evoking a symptom, it should be tested as a single meal on the next four day cycle. If symptoms are evoked, it should be left out for a minimum of six weeks and a maximum of twelve weeks and again introduced into the rotation diet on a trial basis.

3. Some foods combined into a single meal may evoke symptoms when they do not evoke symptoms as a single food or combined with other foods. These types of reactions are best determined on an individual tolerance basis.

4. Occasionally, highly sensitive persons have improved tolerance if exposure to specific foods is kept on a four to seven day rotation combination. Thus the sensitive reactors to wheat, corn, milk and cheese may do well on a basic four day rotation diet for all other foods, but they must eat wheat, corn, milk and cheese at a Saturday or Sunday meal only.

5. When reactions to a large assortment of foods occur, or when the evocation of symptoms is erratic, then the cumulative effect of insecticide residues should be suspected. This can be ruled in or out by (a) test meals of several non-chemically contaminated foods; (b) sublingual provocative tests on an assortment of insecticide sprays used on fruits and vegetables.

6. Some foods within the same family are sufficiently alike, from a chemical standpoint, to bring on symptoms even when spaced two days apart. Examples are wheat, rye, oats and similar gluten-containing foods. Buckwheat contains gluten even though it is not a member of the cereal grain family. However, rice and millet (both of the cereal grain family) do not contain gluten. It is best, therefore, to keep all the gluten-containing cereal grains on a once in four day basis and keep the nongluten cereals on a four day basis two days after the gluten-containing grains. My experience with this system gave satisfactory results.

Maximum restrictive diversified four day rotation diet

DAY FOOD FAMILIES:
1

Rose: Strawberries, blackberries, loganberries, rose hips
Grape: Grapes, raisins
Banana: Bananas, plantains
Apple: Apples
Mulberry: Mulberries, breadfruit
Potato: Potatoes, tomatoes, eggplants, peppers (red and green), chili peppers, paprika, cayenne, ground cherries

Lily: Onions, chives, asparagus
Fungus: Mushrooms, baker's yeast
Beet: Spinach
Mallow: Okra, cottonseed
Grass: Wheat, oats, rye, barley
Buckwheat: Buckwheat, rhubarb
Bovidae: Beef, milk, cheese, yogurt, butter
Mollusca: Scallops, abalones, snails, squid, clams, mussels, oysters
Salt water fish: Mackerel, flounder, anchovies
Walnut: Pecans
Protea: Macadamia nuts
Legume: Peanuts
Flaxseed: Flaxseed
Laurel: Bay leaf, cinnamon
Nutmeg: Nutmeg
Mallow: Maple (maple sugar)
Arrowroot: Arrowroot
Orchid: Vanilla
Sterculia: Cocoa, chocolate
Oil: Peanut, cottonseed
Sweetener: Beet sugar, maple sugar
Tea: Rose hips, strawberry leaf

DAY FOOD FAMILIES:
2

Bird: Chicken, quail, pheasants, eggs of the chicken, quail and pheasant
Plum: Plums, cherries, peaches, almonds
Gourd: Watermelons, pumpkins, cucumbers, acorn squash, pumpkin seeds
Citrus: Oranges, limes
Palm: Coconuts, dates
Papaw: Papaw, papaya, papain
Parsley: Carrots, parsnips, parsley, anise, dill, fennel, cumin, coriander, caraway
Mustard: Watercress, brussels sprouts, collards
Composites: Endive, escarole, artichokes, romaine, safflower, tarragon
Rabbit: Rabbits
Crustaceans: Crabs, crayfish, lobsters

Fresh water fish: Sturgeon, herring, whitefish
Cashew: Cashews
Mint: Basil, sage, horehound, catnip, spearmint
Myrtle: Cloves, allspice
Olive: Olives (black and green)
Oil: Coconut, almond, olive
Sweetener: Date sugar, fructose
Tea: Spearmint, papaya

DAY FOOD FAMILIES:
3

Apple: Pears, quinces
Rose: Raspberries, boysenberries
Heath: Blueberries, huckleberries, cranberries, wintergreen
Gooseberry: Currants, gooseberries
Ebony: Persimmons
Mulberry: Figs
Grass: Corn, rice, millet, cane sorghum
Laurel: Avocadoes, sassafras
Legume: Peas, black-eyed peas, green beans, soybeans, lentils, field peas, kidney beans, lima beans, navy beans, pinto beans, wax beans, carob, alfalfa
Goose foot: Beets, chard, lamb's quarters
Bovidae: Lamb
Suidae: Pork
Salt water fish: Sea herring, cod, sea bass, sea trout, tuna, swordfish, sole
Spurge: Tapioca
Birch: Filberts, hazelnuts
Walnut: English walnuts, hickory nuts, black walnuts
Pepper: Black and white pepper
Lily: Garlic, leeks
Oil: Soybean, avocado, corn
Sweetener: Carob, dextrose, glucose, cane, molasses, sorghum
Tea: Alfalfa, sassafras, raspberry leaf

DAY FOOD FAMILIES:
4

Citrus: Lemons, grapefruits, tangerines, kumquats, citron.
Gourd: Cantaloupes, honeydews, yellow squash, zucchini, squash seeds
Plum: Apricot, nectarines, wild cherries
Cashew: Mangoes, pistachios
Pineapple: Pineapples
Honeysuckle: Elderberries
Morning glory: Sweet potatoes
Mustard: Turnips, radishes, horseradish, Chinese cabbage, broccoli, cauliflower, kale, kohlrabi, rutabaga, mustard
Composites: Lettuce, chicory, dandelion, sunflower seeds
Parsley: Celery, celery seeds
Birds: Turkey, duck, goose, guinea
Crustaceans: Prawns, shrimps
Fresh water fish: Salmon, bass, perch
Beech: Chestnuts
Pedalium: Sesame
Brazil nut: Brazil nuts
Mint: Oregano, savory, peppermint, thyme, marjoram
Nutmeg: Mace
Oil: Sesame, sunflower
Sweetener: Honey
Tea: Peppermint, lemon balm

Minimum restrictive diversified four day rotation diet

1. Foods are kept in families on a four day basis. No member of the family is eaten more frequently than once in four days.

2. *Different foods from the same family can be used on the same day multiple times.*

3. Foods not reacted to can be used multiple times on the same day.

4. If a food has been reacted to, then use it only once in four days after the initial six week or twelve week avoidance period.

This diet is the same as the maximum restrictive diversified four day rotation diet except that it permits multiple meals of members of the same family on the day prescribed for the specific family, providing that no initial reactions to these foods are present on provocative food testing, intradermal serial dilution provocative testing, sublingual (under the tongue) serial dilution provocative testing, or cytotoxic or RAST testing. These different methods of allergy testing are used by various ecological physicians throughout the country.

Limitations to consider when using the minimum restrictive diversified four day rotation diet

1. Maladaptive reactions may develop to foods eaten at different meals during the same day. This is classically due to the cumulative effect of the second or third exposure on the same day. If this occurs, then the food must be left out for six weeks, and when reintroduced into the diet, it should be used once in four days thereafter. Experience with this program reveals that only occasionally do maladaptive reactions develop. Remember, however, the more often specific foods are used, the more likely maladaptive reactions are to occur.

2. Rather than using the same specific foods several times on the same day, it is a safer practice to use other members of the same family at other meals on this same day. Thus wheat, rye or oats could be eaten on the same day but at separate meals. Some prefer a multiple grain breakfast cereal or bread. If this is used, it is preferably used only once, and any member of the cereal grain family it contains should be used neither during the rest of this day nor until the next four day rotation cycle.

Alternative split day minimum restrictive diversified four day rotation diet

This method starts the rotation day with the evening meal. It allows for initially demonstrated nonreactive foods which have been eaten in the evening meal to be eaten also for breakfast the next morning and at noon. Such a diet is for the convenience of the patient and is often appreciated. For most patients who have tried it, there have been good results. It has the inherent danger, however, of multiple exposures of the same food in a twenty-four-hour period which may cumulatively result in an acute reaction.

Four day minimum restricted diversified rotation diet

DAY FOOD FAMILIES:
1

Mulberry: Mulberries, figs, breadfruit
Rose: Strawberries, raspberries, blackberries, dewberries, loganberries, youngberries, boysenberries, rose hips
Grape: All varieties of grapes and raisins, cream of tartar
Potato: Potatoes, tomatoes, eggplants, peppers (red and green), pimentoes, chili peppers, paprika, cayenne, ground cherries
Goose Foot: Beets, spinach, Swiss chard, lamb's quarters (greens)
Composites: Lettuce, chicory, endive, escarole, artichokes, dandelion, tarragon, safflower
Bovidae: Lamb, beef, milk products—butter, cheese, yogurt—goat, deer
Mollusca: Abalone, snails, squid, clams, mussels, oysters, scallops
Spurge: Tapioca
Cashew: Cashews, pistachios, mangoes
Protea: Macadamia nuts
Nutmeg: Nutmeg, mace
Tea: Comfrey, strawberry leaf, raspberry leaf, rose hip
Oil: Safflower
Sweetener: Beet sugar, maple sugar

DAY FOOD FAMILIES:
2

Plum: Plums, cherries, peaches, apricots, nectarines, almonds, wild cherries
Pineapple: Pineapples
Papaw: Papaw, papaya, papain
Myrtle: Guava, clover, allspice, cloves, pimento
Grass: Wheat, corn, rice, oats, barley, rye, wild rice, cane, millet, sorghum, bamboo sprouts
Parsley: Carrots, parsnips, celery, celery seed, celeriac, anise, dill, fennel, cumin, parsley, coriander, caraway
Fungus: Mushrooms and yeast (Brewer's yeast, baker's yeast, etc.)
Mallow: Okra, cottonseed
Bird: All fowl and game birds: chicken, turkey, duck, goose, guineas, pigeon, quail, pheasant, eggs
Salt water fish: Sea herring, anchovies, cod, sea bass, sea trout, mackerel, tuna, swordfish, flounder, sole
Beech: Chestnuts
Subucaya: Brazil nuts
Flaxseed: Flaxseed
Pedalium: Sesame
Orchid: Vanilla
Tea: Papaya tea
Oil: Corn oil, cottonseed oil
Sweetener: Cane sugar (raw), clover honey (if not used on Day 4)
Sterculia: Cocoa, chocolate
Note: Duck, chicken and turkey are in separate families but closely related; they may be eaten every other day or every third day.

DAY FOOD FAMILIES:
3

Apple: Apples, pears, quince
Banana: Bananas, plantains
Arrowroot: Arrowroot
Heath: Blueberries, huckleberries, cranberries, wintergreen
Gooseberry: Currants, gooseberries
Ebony: Persimmons

Legumes: Peas, black-eyed peas, dry beans, green beans, carob, soybeans, lentils, licorice, peanuts, alfalfa
Laurel: Avocadoes, cinnamon, bay leaf, sassafras, cassia buds or bark
Buckwheat: Buckwheat, rhubarb
Lily (onion): Onions, garlic, asparagus, chives, leeks
Crustacea: Crabs, crayfish, lobsters, prawns, shrimp
Suidae: All pork products
Birch: Filberts, hazelnuts
Conifer: Pine nuts
Pepper: Black and white pepper, peppercorn
Tea: Alfalfa tea, sassafras tea
Oil: Soybean, peanut, avocado
Sweetener: Fructose, carob syrup

DAY FOOD FAMILIES:
4

Gourd: Watermelons, cantaloupes, other melons
Citrus: Lemons, oranges, grapefruit, limes, tangerines, kumquats, citron
Honeysuckle: Elderberries
Palm: Coconuts, dates, date sugar
Morning glory: Sweet potatoes
Gourd: Cucumbers, pumpkins, squash, zucchini, acorns, pumpkin or squash seeds
Mustard: Mustard, turnips, radishes, horseradish, watercress, cabbage, kraut, Chinese cabbage, broccoli, cauliflower, brussels sprouts, collards, kale, kohlrabi, rutabaga
Olive: Black or green olives
Fresh water fish: Sturgeon, herring, salmon, whitefish, bass, perch
Walnut: English walnuts, black walnuts, pecans, hickory nuts, butternuts
Mint: Basil, sage, oregano, savory, horehound, catnip, spearmint, peppermint, thyme, marjoram, lemon balm
Tea: Kaffer tea
Oil: Coconut, olive oil, pecan
Sweetener: Date sugar, honey
          Rabbit
          Fowl not used on Day 2

Maximum restrictive seven day diversified rotation diet

This rotation diet is to be used by those who have many severe allergies. Less frequent contacts with food help their systems to clear faster. Only one contact with each food is allowed every seven days, and one must continue to rotate all foods in family groups. Any of the foods listed for a day may be used, but only one contact is permitted with each food. This is best accomplished by using two to five foods at one meal, and not repeating these foods at a following meal.

There are some rare individuals who can eat only one food at each meal, since combinations of any type give rise to symptoms. In such cases, six meals a day can be used, while keeping them on a strict seven day rotation program.

Heating food in oils reduces the absorption rate and hence reduces symptoms. Oils should be rotated. Use corn, safflower, peanut, olive, soy and cottonseed oils, butter, lard and other animal fats, and others. Heating in a Chinese wok is ideal. For those very sensitive persons requiring foods heated in oils, a seven day rotation diet is preferred. Frequent or continual use of foods heated in oil is not recommended, however, since this procedure can raise the patient's free fatty acids and triglycerides. Although there is much medical controversy on the subject of the proper percentage recommendations of fat, carbohydrate and protein to be used in the diet, I believe that the best general program should contain 10 to 20 percent protein, 10 to 15 percent fat and 70 to 80 percent complex carbohydrates (unrefined) per week. These percentages are based on total caloric intake. At the present time, there is considerable debate in medical circles about the value of various percentages of dietary fat, protein and carbohydrates. Nathan Pritikin concludes from the medical literature that 10 percent fat, 10 percent protein, and 80 percent complex carbohydrate as total calories provides the optimum ratio for reversal of and protection from arteriosclerosis when this is also accompanied by systematic exercise. This evidence serves as a valuable guideline. It should be understood that these percentages were arrived at without benefit of laboratory demonstration of individual nutritional needs, and without benefit of nutritional supplementation. Supplementary vitamin C and pyridoxine would serve as additional protection against the inflammation leading to arthromatos plaque formation, irrespective of percentages of carbohydrates, proteins or fats. A practical consideration would likely be in the range of 10 to 15 percent fat, 10 to 20 percent protein, 70 to 80 percent complex carbohydrates, as total calories, with infrequent use of simple sugars. Extensive research needs yet to be done in this area.

Maximum restrictive seven day diversified rotation diet

DAY FOOD FAMILIES:
1

Apple: Apples, pears, quince
Mulberry: Mulberries, figs, breadfruit
Honeysuckle: Elderberries
Olives: Black or green olives
Gooseberry: Currants, gooseberries
Potato: Potatoes, tomatoes, eggplants, peppers (red and green), chili peppers, paprika, cayenne
Lily: Onions, garlic, asparagus, chives, leeks
Grass: Wheat, corn, rice, oats, barley, rye, wild rice, cane, millet, sorghum, bamboo sprouts
Buckwheat: Buckwheat, rhubarb
Bovidae: Milk products, butter, cheese, yogurt, beef and pure beef products, lamb
Mint: Basil, savory, sage, oregano, horehound, catnip, spearmint, peppermint, thyme, marjoram, lemon balm
Tea: Elder, mint, catnip
Oil: Olive, corn, 100 percent corn oil margarine, butter

Juices: Juices may be made and used without adding sweeteners from the following:
Fruits: any listed above in any combination desired
Vegetables: any listed above in any combination desired

DAY FOOD FAMILIES:
2

Citrus: Lemons, oranges, kumquats, citron, grapefruits, limes, tangerines
Parsley: Carrots, celeriac, parsley, anise, parsnips, celery, celery seed, dill, cumin, coriander, caraway, fennel
Pepper: White pepper
Nutmeg: Mace
Walnut: English walnuts, black walnuts, pecans, hickory nuts, butternuts
Bird: Chicken, goose, quail and their eggs
Tea: Comfrey tea, comfrey greens, fennel
Oil: Fat from any bird listed above
Oil from any nut listed above
Sweetener: Orange honey, used sparingly
Juices: Juices may be made and used without added
sweeteners from the following:
Fruits: any listed above in any combination desired
Vegetables: any listed above in any combination
desired

DAY FOOD FAMILIES:
3

Grape: All varieties of grapes and raisins
Rose: Strawberries, raspberries, blackberries, dewberries, loganberries, youngberries, boysenberries, rose hips
Legumes: Pea, black-eyed peas, dry beans, string beans, carob, soybeans, lentils, licorice, peanuts, alfalfa
Flaxseed: Flaxseed
Suidae: All pork products
Arrowroot: Arrowroot
Tea: Alfalfa tea, rose hip tea
Oil: Peanut or soy
Sweetener: Carob syrup, used sparingly, clover honey (if honey not used on any other day)

Juices: Juices may be made and used without added sweeteners, from the following:
Fruits: any listed above in any combination desired
Vegetables: any listed above in any combination desired

DAY FOOD FAMILIES:
4

Heath: Blueberries, huckleberries, cranberries, wintergreen
May apple: May apples
Papaw: Papaw, papaya, papain
Composite: Lettuce, chicory, endive, escarole, artichoke, dandelion, sunflower seeds, tarragon, oyster plant (salsify), celtuse
Morning glory: Sweet potatoes (not yams)
Laurel: Avocado, cinnamon, bay leaf, sassafras, cassia buds or bark
Protea: Macadamia nuts
Beech: Chestnuts
Orchid: Vanilla
Fungus: Mushrooms and yeast
Salt water fish: Sea herring, anchovies, cod, sea bass, sea trout, mackerel, tuna, swordfish, flounder, sole
Oil: Avocado
Tea: Sassafras tea, papaya
Spurge: Tapioca
Juices: Juices may be made and used without added sweeteners from the following:
Fruits: any listed above in any combination desired
Vegetables: any listed above in any combination desired

DAY FOOD FAMILIES:
5

Pineapple: Pineapples
Gourd: Watermelons, cucumbers, cantaloupes, pumpkins, squash (all varieties), other melons, zucchini, summer squash
Purslane: Purslane, New Zealand spinach greens

Mallow: Okra, cottonseed
Cashew: Cashews, pistachios, mango
Pedalium: Sesame
Mollusca: Abalone, snails, squid, clams, mussels, oysters, scallops
Crustacea: Crabs, crayfish, lobsters, prawns, shrimp
Tea: Fenugreek
Oil: Cottonseed, sesame
Juices: Juices may be made and used without added sweeteners from the following:
Fruits: any listed above in any combination desired
Vegetables: any listed above in any combination desired

DAY FOOD FAMILIES:
6

Banana: Bananas, plantains, arrowroot (musa)
Pomegranate: Pomegranates
Ebony: Persimmons
Palm: Coconuts, dates, date sugar, sago, palm cabbage
Pepper: Black pepper, peppercorns
Nutmeg: Nutmeg
Beet: Beets, chard, spinach, lamb's quarters (greens)
Birch: Filberts, hazelnuts
Bird: Turkey, duck, pigeon, pheasant and their eggs
Oil: Coconut oil and fat from any bird listed above
Sweetener: Date sugar or beet sugar (use sparingly)
Juices: Juices may be added and used without added sweeteners from the following:
Fruits: any listed above in any combination desired
Vegetables: any listed above in any combination desired

DAY FOOD FAMILIES:
7

Plum: Plums, cherries, peaches, apricots, nectarines, almonds, wild cherries, also small amounts of any natural dried version of fruit listed above
Mustard: Mustard, turnips, radishes, horseradish, watercress,

cabbage, kraut, Chinese cabbage, broccoli, cauliflower,
brussels sprouts, collards, kale, kohlrabi, rutabaga
Yam: Yams, Chinese potatoes
Subucaya: Brazil nuts
Conifer: Pine nuts
Oil: Safflower
Tea: Safflower, mate
Bovidae: Lamb
Sweetener: Buckwheat, safflower and sage honey, if honey is
not used on any other day
Juices: Juices may be made and used without added sweeten-
ers from the following:
Fruits: any listed above in any combination desired
Vegetables: any listed above in any combination
desired

Special tips for using the rotation diet

HOW TO SWITCH FOOD FAMILIES

In the preceding pages, we have presented the food families
and have divided them on a four day diet and a seven day
diet. If you would like a food on a different day from where
we placed it, you may switch the entire family to another
day. When you have the food family on the day you prefer,
leave it on that day so that the food is not eaten more
often than prescribed.

SUBSTITUTES FOR COMMON FOODS

Margarine: Use the oil of the day, mix in the blender with
nuts and seasonings. This can be used to top vegetables.

Beverages: Use the spices of the day, i.e., mace, nutmeg,
anise, cinnamon, clove, etc., and brew as a tea, mix half and half
with fruit juices. Serve iced or hot.

Egg: Use 8 oz. dried apricots soaked until soft in two cups
water and mix in blender. A generous tablespoon of this mixture
is equal to one egg in a dough mixture. Another substitute is one
cup ground flaxseed boiled three minutes in three cups water. Stir

constantly. Keep in closed jar in refrigerator. One tablespoon equals one egg. There are also commercial egg replacers on the market.

Milk: Mix 2 oz. almonds or pine nuts, or 1 teaspoon sesame seeds with 1 teaspoon honey and 1 cup of water in a blender for use in recipes. Also a commercial soya milk product is available.

Salad dressings: Use ascorbic acid (vitamin C), one table-spoon to one cup water, as a substitute for vinegar in salad dressings. Combine vitamin C mixture, oil of the day, salt and spices of the day to give you a great variety of dressings. Avocadoes, tomatoes, onions, celery and other vegetables and cheeses can be added as the day allows.

Purposeful violation of diversified rotation diet

When a rotation is successfully established, it is possible occasionally to eat a single meal of multiple foods without respect to rotation. It is best to reserve this as a treat for special occasions once a month or so. Alcohol should not be used with this meal as it will multiply by four the chances of a reaction occurring. When needed, a considerable degree of protection from maladaptive reactions to these special occasion meals can be achieved by the following, taken singly or as a total program:

1. One hour ahead of the meal, take 4 grams of sodium ascorbate (vitamin C).

2. One hour ahead of the meal, take five 350 mg pancreas enzyme capsules or tablets. Some do better by adding three to five 100 mg bromelain tablets to this.

3. One hour ahead of the meal, take 5 to 15 grams of free amino acids.

4. Immediately before the meal, take sublingually (under the tongue) 1250 to 2500 units of heparin. Heparin sublingually placed in a dose ranging from 1250 to 2500 units can serve as a great protection against inflammatory allergic reactions. This can be given ten to fifteen minutes ahead of a meal and, if a reaction to a meal occurs, it can be used immediately to help reduce the

symptoms. It is simple for people to carry heparin with them
and have it readily available for sublingual use. This amount of
heparin is considerably below the anticoagulant doses for which
heparin has been placed on the market but it does serve as a good
anti-inflammatory agent at this level. Heparin or the other
enzymes can also be used as a protection against petrochemical
hydrocarbons during shopping, an inadvertent exposure to car
exhaust and so forth. It is not wise to use these anti-inflammatory
agents to try to ride through a chronic exposure where avoidance and spacing of contact can be arranged but they do serve a
valuable purpose in making life liveable during the occasional
exposure that cannot be avoided.

5. With the meal, take 500 mg pyridoxine, 100–500 mg
riboflavin, 500 mg pantothenic acid.

6. At the end of the meal, take 1 pancreas enzyme capsule
or tablet. Some do well to add one 100 mg bromelain tablet to
this.

7. Thirty to sixty minutes after the end of the meal, take 1 to
5 pancreas enzyme capsules or tablets. Some do well to add 1 to
100 mg bromelain tablets to this.

8. Thirty to sixty minutes after the end of the meal, take 10 to
20 gm sodium bicarbonate or sodium and potassium bicarbonate
(3:1 ratio).

9. If any symptoms develop after the meal, take 2500 units
heparin sublingually. Also, the pancreas enzymes and bicarbonate can be taken sooner than the 30 to 60 minute period if
symptoms occur. A much more detailed discussion on the use of
this type of "nutrient therapy" will be forthcoming in subsequent
chapters.

Chemically contaminated food

Inherently many foods contain toxins which require detoxification by the liver or other metabolic means such as by
vitamin C, oxygenation, and the like. Molds producing toxins
and/or maladaptive allergies or allergic-like reactions are
frequent in foods. In recent years manufacturers have
added insecticide residues to fruits and vegetables with the

resultant contamination of meats and milk. This added burden of detoxification and potential maladaptive reactions hastens the degenerative disease process. Ideally toxins should be as low as possible in our foods and water supply. Some people, however, are so sensitive and have such a low level of detoxifying ability that of necessity they must use foods and water that are not chemically contaminated. Theron G. Randolph, M.D., and several others who have followed his lead have demonstrated the value of initially testing with chemically noncontaminated foods and then later selectively testing nonreactive foods contaminated with insecticides. Marshall Mandell, M.D., has demonstrated the value of sublingual provocative testing to determine maladaptive reactions to insecticide residues.

Summary

The latter part of the nineteenth century and the early part of the twentieth brought to medicine a significant array of ecologic facts which not only led to some valuable present-day health measures but also helped to develop the fields of bacteriology and allergy. Before the ecologic orientation had made its full contribution, however, such body centered areas as pathology and pharmacology (drugs) were giving promise of rapid cure and/or quick symptomatic relief. The promise of such treatment methods tended to eclipse the significance of ecologic facts. Recently a resurgence of interest in human ecology has been occurring due to the developing consciousness of how the ever increasing pollution of our entire environment is adversely influencing man. Another factor that is causing this trend is the clinically demonstrated position which categorically proves that frequently eaten foods and commonly met chemicals are capable of adversely altering central nervous system functions.

The ecologic method of comprehensive environmental control provides for a specific period of avoidance of all possible incriminating substances. Such a program, in many cases, actually "turns off" by the fourth day the chronic physical or mental illness. The illness is turned back on by precipitating an acute reaction upon a single exposure to a food or chemical. In this way, induction evidence of symptom causes is clearly demonstrated; we can, therefore, at least believe what we see. This evidence leads to the conclusion that the basic organic driving forces behind many chronic physical and mental illnesses are addictive reactions to frequently eaten foods and commonly met chemicals. After one has been exposed to all the ecologic facts presented in this book, the significant message—that any food and/or chemical is capable of maintaining chronic physical and mental reactions in susceptible persons, and that following a four to seven day period in which incriminating food and chemicals are faithfully avoided, there is clinical improvement in chronic symptoms—will, I hope, become obvious. The sad truth is, however, that we Americans are eating our foods with a frequency that is beyond our biological capacity to handle in a healthy way. After seeing hundreds of clinical cases, it has become increasingly clear to us that if people were taught to rotate their foods, many chronic physical and mental illnesses would be prevented. Not only can this rotation program provide a frequency contact which the human organism can metabolically handle and for which it was designed, it can also materially improve the nutritional state of each and every one of us due to the fact that we are contacting a desirably larger assortment of foods in a properly managed four day rotation diet.

One can say that maladaptive reactions and their counterpart, addiction, along with nutritional deficiency and infection, are the building blocks from which chronic diseases are built. It matters not with which one of these we start; the others will soon follow. Of these three, the most important beginning point of many illnesses, as far as our clinical evidence reveals, is that of allergy-addiction, with nutritional deficiency and infection following closely.

It cannot be overemphasized that a four or more day rotation of foods (especially symptom incriminated foods) is of prime importance when attempting to ecologically control the addictive state. But it would certainly be wrong to conclude that a rotation diet alone is the cure-all of physical and mental illness. Nutrients in proper amounts and types can help prevent the majority of maladaptive reactions to foods and/or chemicals. Intravenous and oral administration of nutrients have been demonstrated clinically to be capable of preventing maladaptive food and chemical reactions. The ideal form of treatment, therefore, combines both the ecological and the orthomolecular treatment methodologies. In order that we can begin to understand the fundamentals of the physical and mental disease process, let us now switch emphasis from food-chemical (ecological) management to nutritional management. An in-depth understanding of both of these important aspects of treatment is necessary.

SUGGESTED READING

1. Philpott, W. H., Nielsen, R. and Pierson, V. 1976. Four-day rotation of foods according to families. *In Clinical Ecology.* Dickey, L. D., ed. Springfield IL: Charles C. Thomas, pp. 472–486.

2. Pritikin, N. 1979. *The Pritikin Diet and Exercise Program.* New York: Grosset and Dunlap.

3. Randolph, T. G. 1956. The descriptive features of food addiction: addictive eating and drinking. *Alcohol Studies* 17:198.

4. Rinkel, H. J., Randolph, T. S. and Zeller, M. 1951. *Food Allergy.* Springfield, IL.: Charles C. Thomas.

CHAPTER FIVE

The importance of fiber in the diabetic diet

Until recently, the study of how plant fibers influence gastrointestinal physiology and the absorption of many different yet important nutrients had been seriously neglected by most scientists and physicians. During a large part of this century, scientific attention concentrated on the interactions of specific vitamins, minerals, proteins, fats or carbohydrates, but plant fibers, considered by most to be nonnutritive in value, had not undergone such a rigorous scientific evaluation. In the last five to ten years, however, empirical experimentation has clearly demonstrated the fact that fiber does indeed play a significant role in the proper absorption, digestion and metabolism of *all* our food and nutrients contained therein.

In order to appreciate how important fiber is in the normal as well as diabetic diet, we must first define some terms. Plant fiber is that portion of the plant which is not digested in the human small intestine. While most fibers are structural components of plant cell walls, some fibers (i.e., gums) are manufactured by the plant to serve specific functions, while others (i.e., guar) are stored by the plant to meet future energy needs. There are two basic types of plant fibers, namely those which are soluble in water and those which are not.

The three major categories of soluble fibers are: pectins, gums and mucilages, and polysaccharides. Pectins, which are structural components of plant cell walls, are found predominantly in fruits and contribute to over 40 percent of the fruits' fiber. Gums and mucilages, on the other hand, are not structural in nature, but rather serve specific functions for the plant. Often you will discover gums at sites of injury and they are sticky in nature. Polysaccharides are known for their water absorbing and binding characteristics, and are used as stored energy sources by most plants. The three major categories of insoluble fibers are cellulose, hemicellulose and lignin. Cellulose, the most well known form of plant fiber, represents over 25 percent of the plant fiber content of many grains, vegetables and fruits. Hemicellulose, a form of fiber structurally similar to cellulose, composes 50 to 70 percent of the plant fiber in grains, vegetables and fruits. The lignins, representing only 10 percent of the total plant fiber, are best known for their extreme resistance to human digestion.

But what does all this talk have to do specifically with the etiology of diabetes? To answer this very important question, we must first look at some statistical data which, while demonstrating only association and not a cause and effect relationship, offers a consistent hypothesis that fiber, or more accurately the lack of fiber, may be an important component in the dietary cause of diabetes. As far back as 1960, a researcher named Trowell[1] developed a hypothesis that the high fiber diet of the black villagers in rural Africa might protect them from diabetes. As expected, he discovered that the incidence of diabetes was much lower with the rural villagers who had an extremely high intake of plant fiber, as compared to the urban dwellers who had both a low fiber intake and a much higher prevalence of diabetes. But what is even more noteworthy is the fact that most of the epidemiological studies done by other researchers confirmed Trowell's original hypothesis. The incidence of

diabetes is very low, for example, with the Transvaal
Bantu and the Yemenite Jews, both of whom have a high
intake of complex carbohydrates and plant fiber; however,
the incidence of diabetes has increased dramatically in both
groups within the last ten to twenty years after they ate
refined flour and a low fiber diet.[2] Moreover, if you compare
the low incidence of diabetes (2 percent) in East Pakistan,
where 83 percent of calories come from the dietary intake of
complex carbohydrates (i.e., vegetables, fruits, grains,
legumes), and thus high fiber foods, with the very high
incidence of diabetes (17 percent) in Pennsylvania, where
less than 35 percent of calories come from high fiber foods,
you begin to see the possibility that diabetes may indeed
be inversely correlated with the intake of plant fiber.

Obviously, statistical data only proves association of
facts; it does not prove causation. But if one can combine
statistical association with similar evidence received from
clinical-empirical observations, then a valid case for the
need of fiber in our diet as a protective agent against
diabetes can be made. This, of course, is difficult to do, but
clinical scientists have clearly demonstrated by experimentation that fiber does significantly protect one against the
killer disease known as diabetes. Let us now, therefore,
examine in an in-depth fashion some of this experimental
data.

Jenkins[3] was one of the first researchers to prove that
when carbohydrates are eaten with certain plant fibers,
less high blood sugar (hyperglycemia) results as to compared to when carbohydrates are eaten by themselves.
More specifically, when he fed individuals without diabetes
a 50 gram glucose load with and without fiber, he discovered that blood glucose levels after glucose and guar were
significantly lower than values after glucose alone. He also
fed large test meals (i.e., 106 grams carbohydrates, 9.6 grams
protein, 17.8 grams fat) with and without fiber to normal
individuals and discovered again that blood sugar levels
after the meal were much lower in the individuals receiving additional guar supplementation than in those who did
not.

These important clinical experiments demonstrating the importance of plant fiber and carbohydrate tolerance were also run on patients suffering from chemical diabetes. Jenkins again discovered that when similar test meals were fed to diabetics, the elevation of blood sugar levels as well as serum insulin levels was substantially less after the meals with guar as compared to the meals without guar. Another researcher named Monnier[4] found results similar to Jenkins's. In his experiments with diabetic individuals he found hyperglycemia to be noticeably less after glucose and pectin as compared to glucose alone. It is safe to conclude, therefore, that both the studies with normal individuals and those with diabetic individuals unequivocally prove that soluble plant fibers decreased postmeal blood sugar and serum insulin levels.

Numerous studies have shown the long term beneficial effects that plant fiber has on glucose metabolism. Broadribb,[5] for example, has reported that when patients with diverticula disease were given about 24 grams of wheat bran daily for six months, hyperglycemia levels were much lower than those reported before the bran supplementation program began. Anderson[6] has reported that a diet of high complex carbohydrates (i.e., vegetables, legumes, fruits) and thus high fiber has had very favorable effects on patients with diabetes. The experimental diet consisted of about 60 percent complex carbohydrate, 20 percent protein and 20 percent fat, with about 25 grams of plant fiber per 1,000 calories of food. During the twenty-one months in which eleven diabetic patients maintained this diet, their insulin, glucose, cholesterol and triglyceride levels were all significantly lower. Douglass[7] carried this previous experiment a step further and reported that insulin doses could be lowered in patients placed on a "raw diet" containing large amounts of uncooked vegetables, seeds, nuts and fruits. Such a diet, of course, contains large quantities of plant fibers in their natural form.

One of the most comprehensive studies done to date from the relationship of high carbohydrate (high in nutrients and fiber) diet and diabetes was done by J. W. Ander-

son. The evidence as compiled, based on clinical testing,
clearly points to the fact that a high complex carbohydrate
diet, which obciously supplies a rich abundance of not
only fiber but also vitamins, minerals, amino acids and trace
elements—all extremely important to the diabetic, as
shown in Chapters five through nine—has a very beneficial
effect on patients suffering from diabetes. Such a diet
maintained over sixteen days actually reduced the insulin
requirements of his experimental diabetic subjects. Writes
Anderson:

*The short-term effects of high-carbohydrate, high-fiber (HCF)
diets on lean individuals with diabetes have been further examined
in detail. On a metabolic ward, patients received weight-
maintaining controlled diets (43 percent of energy from carbohy-*

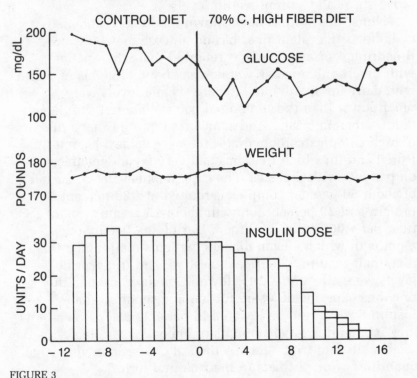

FIGURE 3

Response to High-carbohydrate, High-fiber (HCF) Diet.

*This man was fed the control and HCF diets as described by Anderson
and Ward.*

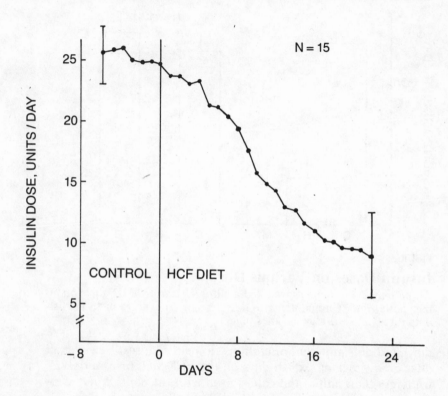

FIGURE 4

Changes in Insulin Doses on Control and HCF Diets.

Body weights of these lean men were maintained constant throughout these studies. (From the studies of Anderson and colleagues.)

drate, 19 percent protein, 38 percent fat with 12 grams plant
fiber per 1,000 calories) for six to eleven days followed by
weight-maintaining HCF diets (70 percent carbohydrate, 19
percent protein, 11 percent fat with 36 grams plant fiber per 1,000
calories) for twelve to twenty-eight days. All diets consisted of
natural foods which are available in most grocery stores. The high
level of fiber intake was achieved by using high-fiber foods such
as whole grain and bran products, legumes, and vegetables. The
response of a represented patient is presented in figure 3. Figure
4 shows the time course of changes in insulin doses when
constant body weights and plasma glucose concentrations were
maintained. Patients on controlled diets for a minimum of eight

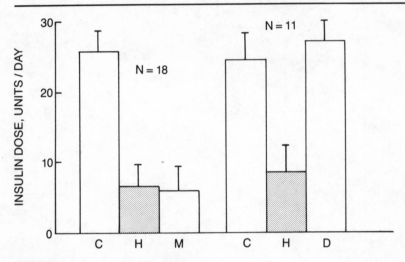

FIGURE 5

Insulin Doses on Various Diets.

*All patients with diabetes were fed control (C) and HCF (H) diets on a
metabolic ward. On maintenance (M) diets for an average of 16 mo as
outpatients, insulin doses were stable.*

*days had no significant alterations in insulin doses. However,
after an average of sixteen days on the HCF diet, insulin doses
were less than half of the values used with the control diet. The
changes in insulin doses on HCF diets for thirty patients are
summarized in figure 5.[8]*

It is important to briefly note that water soluble plant fibers
also lower cholesterol and triglyceride levels. Anderson[9]
has found that pectin, guar and extracts of specific legumes
have had significant powers of lowering cholesterol in
humans. In experiments done on animals, Anderson has
found that certain polysaccharides extracted from legumes
can lower cholesterol levels by as much as 80 percent in
rats. Also, studies done by Anderson[10] indicate that diets
high in plant fiber can simultaneously lower not only
cholesterol but triglyceride levels. In his usual competent
and extremely thorough manner, Anderson has shown a 63
percent reduction of triglyceride levels in experimental
subjects maintained on a high complex carbohydrate high
fiber diet. Conversely, fasting serum triglyceride values

actually rose in patients fed high carbohydrate *low fiber* diets. Based on these clinical findings, Anderson concludes, "since hypertriglyceridemia and hypercholesterolemia are fairly common in persons with diabetes, an increase in plant fiber intake may be beneficial for certain patients."[11] Such a statement is obviously true for those individuals currently suffering from the cardiovascular complications (high cholesterol) and high triglyceride so commonly associated with diabetes.

In summary, based on the preceding clinical studies as well as on the evidence that will be forthcoming in subsequent chapters, it is accurate to conclude that an increase in consumption of such high fiber foods as whole grains, vegetables, legumes, seeds and fruits—preferably in their raw state—will benefit most people to a significant degree of improvement in their health. This is especially true for those suffering from diabetes and its cardiovascular complications.

In addition to a deficiency of fiber in the diet, allergic or otherwise maladaptive reactions to foods and chemicals should also be considered as etiological possibilities for causing such bowel related problems as constipation, diarrhea, spastic colon, colitis and so forth. The basic corrective treatment for these conditions is to discover the foods and/or chemicals that evoke these symptoms. An initial avoidance for three months and later a four to seven day spacing of these symptom incriminating substances usually provide a symptom-free state. Obviously, water retention in the colon and bulk from fiber content in foods are major factors in bowel control once the symptom incriminating foods have been isolated and avoided. Also, optimum vitamin C as well as acidophilus bacteria supplementation combined with adequate fluid intake are other essential factors in achieving healthy colon function.

Ascorbate, preferably as ascorbic acid (vitamin C), or sodium ascorbate should be taken in adequate amounts to retain sufficient water in the colon and thus keep the stool both soft and formed. For those adults having bowel-related problems, this usually requires four grams and sometimes more three times a day. Vitamin C should be increased until desired bowel consistency is achieved. This program also serves the purpose of detoxifying bacterial toxins formed in the colon and encourages a normal bacterial flora to flourish. It is, therefore, better to use such a nonirritating ascorbate fluid retention program of treatment than irritative laxatives. If too much ascorbate is taken, diarrhea might occur. When this happens, simply reduce the ascorbate until the diarrhea disappears. All dose requirements must be determined on an individual basis and preferably under the supervision of a trained Bio-Ecologic physician.

Our daily stools should be formed, soft and have sufficient fiber to float in water. Each day should be planned to contain adequate fiber in the diet. Fiber sources, however, should be rotated on a four day basis in keeping with the four day diversified rotation diet. Fiber sources from foods that initially evoked allergic symptoms should not be used for the first three months and, when reintroduced into the diet, should be used only once in four days.

Good bowel control requires fiber sources from a wide assortment of foods. Fruits such as apples, pears and so forth should be eaten with skins when possible. Potatoes should be eaten with skins. Cereal grains should be eaten as whole grain foods. Alfalfa tablets are also a good source of fiber and, if not maladaptively reacted to, should be used on the suitable day of rotation by taking ten tablets three times a day. Psyllium husks and milled comfrey are excellent fiber sources and can be taken as one to three teaspoons three times a day, once every four days in rotation. More common fiber sources to consider are: wheat bran, wheat germ, rice polishings, greens of many types, celery, pineapple and so forth. It is a wise policy to freeze vegetables so they are available the year around; it is also preferable to steam rather than to boil them in the cooking process.

As a final note, eight to ten glasses of fluids besides the water normally contained in your foods is necessary for adequate water to be available for the colon. If fruit or vegetable juices are your choices of liquids, make sure you rotate them on at least a four day basis.

REFERENCES

1. Trowell, H. 1960. *Non-infective Disease in Africa*. London: Edward Arnold.

2. West, K. M. and Kalbfleisch, J. M. 1971. influence of nutritional factors on prevalence of diabetes. *Diabetes* 20:99–108.

3. Jenkins, D. J. 1978. Dietary fibers and glucose tolerance. *British Medical Journal* 1:1392–1394.

4. Monnier, L. 1978. Influence of indigestible fibers on glucose tolerance. *Diabetes Care* 1:83–88.

5. Broadribb, A. 1976. Diverticular disease: three studies. *British Medical Journal* 2:424–430.

6. Anderson, J. W. 1979. High carbohydrate, high fiber diets for patients with diabetes. *Proceedings of Fourth International Symposium of Early Diabetes*. New York: Plenum Press.

7. Douglass, J. M. 1975. Raw diet and insulin requirements. *Annals of Internal Medicine* 82:61–62.

8. Anderson, J. W. July–August 1979. Fiber and diabetes. *Diabetes Care* 2:4.

9. _____. 1979. Plant fiber, carbohydrate and lipid metabolism. *American Journal of Clinical Nutrition* 32:346–363.

10. _____. 1978. Triglyceride lowering effects of high fiber diets. *Clinical Research* 27:548A.

11. _____. 1979. Fiber and diabetes.

CHAPTER SIX

Vitamin B6, cardiovascular complications and cholesterol

Arteriosclerotic heart disease is the greatest single cause of death in the United States today. People with diabetes are six times more likely to suffer arteriosclerotic related heart attacks and strokes than are people without diabetes.
These figures are a result of research studies done by the U.S. Public Health Service, the National Institute of Health, the American Heart Association, the American Diabetes Association and by private insurance companies. In fact, the statistical association existing between diabetes and cardiovascular and cerebrovascular disease is so close that many physicians are beginning to ask whether the basic arteriosclerotic process that leads to heart attacks and strokes is not in reality the diabetic disease process itself.
"The name of the game in diabetes research," writes Bertrand E. Lowenstein, M.D., "is preventing the vascular and neurological complications of diabetes. The growing portion of the medical profession now realizes that neither insulin, oral anti-diabetic agents, nor contemporary diet programs can do this job. Diabetes remains an unbridled

killer and maimer, and the notion that it is controllable remains a myth."[1] Indeed, arteriosclerosis and diabetes may be, in reality, two sides of the same metabolic coin. For the diabetic disease process alters natural chemical functions so dramatically as to actually cause damage to certain physical structures inside the blood vessels, especially in the microscopic blood vessels throughout the body. When the blood vessels of the heart are affected by this process, deposits of metabolic debris eventually clog up some of the coronary vessels, closing them off to proper circulation; the result is a heart attack. If the blood vessels that supply the brain are affected by the same process, the result of course is a stroke. Other areas of the body besides the coronary and cerebral vessels that can be affected by this process are the retinas of the eyes, the capillaries of the kidney, and capillaries of the lower legs, especially the feet. When the eyes are afflicted, the condition is known as diabetic retinopathy or retinitis. When the kidney is afflicted, the disease is nephropathy. Gangrene occurs when the lower legs and feet are afflicted. All of these vascular problems associated with diabetes are in reality based, as we shall see, upon nutritional deficiencies created by the diabetic disease process.

An entire specialty field in medicine known as Bio-Ecologic Medicine has developed a specific treatment modality precisely designed to eliminate these nutritional complications of diabetes. That is, Bio-Ecologic Medicine approaches the problems of diabetes and arteriosclerosis with the assumption that the human body is a wonderful and incredible biochemical machine in which there are literally thousands of chemical and biochemical reactions taking place every microsecond. Each reaction requires certain optimum conditions and the right amounts of certain chemical substances for maximum benefit. More specifically, Bio-Ecologic Medicine is based on the idea that an ideal optimal environment for each cell of our bodies includes not only an ample supply of water and oxygen and a suitable ambient temperature but also a team of about forty nutrients, all of which must be combined in the right proportions in order to work together toward the ideal of perfect health. These forty some nutrients include a list of vitamins, minerals, trace elements and amino acids. If any of these substances are not present in the correct amounts, abnormal and alternative pathways result.

It is further recognized by those who practice Bio-Ecologic Medicine that the cells of our bodies usually have to tolerate environments which fall considerably short of the ideal. And even if just the right assortment of nutrients is supplied to the body, the digestion, absorption and transportation of these nutrients is not an automatic process. This, of course, implies that if any link in the biochemical chain is weak or missing, the cells will be inadequately supplied and ill health will quickly follow. The weak link might be something like an iron or calcium deficiency, a tyrosine (amino acid) deficiency, a vitamin B6 or vitamin C deficiency, an improper absorption or digestion of these nutrients, or deficiencies of a trace mineral like selenium or chromium, or any number of other situations. The result of any of these deficiencies plus the possibility of an almost infinite number of other deficiencies is always the same: an impoverished biochemical environment which inevitably leads to functional impairment.

Another idea used by those practicing Bio-Ecologic Medicine is the fact that nutritional needs among individuals are distinctively different for each and every person alive. Hence, there can be no general program that everyone can or must follow. Each person's biochemical uniqueness must be taken into account. We cannot, for example, safely assume that furnishing a high quality, protein rich diet will provide adequate amounts of all the essential amino acids necessary for optimum health. There are numerous digestive enzymes, as we have seen, which break down proteins into amino acids, some of which might be functioning well in certain people, and in others not at all. Obviously, if the former is the case, there should be an adequate supply of amino acids in the blood; if the latter is true, the supply will be deficient. As for vitamins,

minerals and trace elements, each individual's unique
need levels are even more distinctive. In fact, vitamin
tolerance levels may vary as much as a thousandfold
among patients in our clinic.

Dr. Linus Pauling defined Orthomolecular Medicine as
that discipline which "varies the concentration of substances
(i.e., vitamins, minerals, trace elements, amino acids,
hormones and enzymes, etc.) normally present in the human
body in the treatment of diseases of all kinds." Bio-Ecologic
physicians insist that the battle against disease, and of
course this includes diabetes and arteriosclerosis, should
always be with weapons (nutrients) which are most
similar to nature's own biological weapons. If we are sick
in any way, the Bio-Ecologic view is that the cells of our
bodies are ailing because they are being inadequately
provisioned with the proper nutrients they need for correct
metabolism and health. We have already pointed out that,
should a cell become deficient in one or a group of
nutrients, its entire function will be seriously impaired.
And if you multiply one deranged cell by a few hundred
million, then tissues and organs—even the pancreas—are
affected, and one experiences what modern medicine calls
degenerative disease.

We will begin our examination of Bio-Ecologic treatment
of the degenerative diseases named diabetes and arteriosclerosis by discussing generally all the major vitamins
needed for optimum health. We will then focus more
specifically on just a few of these vitamins, so as to present
a more detailed explanation of their function in the
treatment of these disorders. In later chapters, we will
examine certain major minerals and trace elements to see
the relationships existing between the proper balance of
these "essential nutrients" and optimum health.

Orthomolecular treatment, vitamins and diabetes

The name vitamin comes from vita (life), plus amine
(chemical compounds originally thought to be present in

vitamins). Vitamins are not alien substances to our body as are drugs; rather, they are organic substances which are essential for the proper functioning of human beings as well as animals. They should never be thought of as miraculous cure-alls. Instead, they are essential nutrients, and physical as well as mental illness will be the result when there are deficiencies of these chemicals in the human body. Vitamins are present in minute quantities in many foods. Basically there are two types of vitamins: fat soluble, and water soluble. Fat soluble vitamins such as A, D, E, and K are soluble in ethanol (alcohol), and are associated with lipids (fat) of natural foods. They are more easily stored within the body. All B-complex vitamins (B1, B2, B3, B5, B6, and B12), vitamin C, biotin, folic acid and para-amino-benzoic acid are water soluble vitamins. Water soluble vitamins are easily lost by the body in the urine. Chemically speaking, all of the above mentioned vitamins are distinctively different. Table 6.1 lists some of their general functions, therapeutic uses and dietary sources.

Table 6.1*

Vitamin	Function & uses	Dietary sources
A	Good vision, healthy skin and hair, prevention of acne.	Butter, cod liver oil, milk, egg, liver, kidney, carrots, yellow fruits, dark green fruits and vegetables
B1 (thiamine)	Prevents beriberi, necessary for proper functioning of nervous system, heart and carbohydrate metabolism. Used for correcting insomnia, constipation, irritability and loss of appetite.	Brewer's yeast, liver, heart, kidney, meat, leafy green vegetables, egg yolk, legumes, nuts, milk, whole grains and blackstrap molasses

*Fat soluble group of vitamins such as A, D, E and K cannot be absorbed from the intestine in the absence of bile. The presence of vitamin antimetabolites and antagonists (such as antibiotics) in diet or body fluid greatly reduces their potency, resulting in deficiency. Cooking (heat) destroys vitamins B1, B2, B3, B6 and biotin.

Vitamin	Function & uses	Dietary sources
B2 (riboflavin)	Deficiency may result in localized seborrheic dermatitis of the face, magenta tongue, cheilosis. Helps light-sensitive eyes.	Same as for B1
B3 (niacin)	Carbohydrate metabolism, circulatory system, applications include mental fatigue, hyperlipidemia, dermatitis, weakness, abdominal pains, schizophrenia.	Same as for B1, plus salmon
B5 (pantothenic acid)	A constituent of coenzyme A, which is essential to several fundamental reactions in metabolism. Deficiency produces profound effect on the adrenal gland, synthesis of cholesterol, steroid hormones, utilization of carbohydrate, fat and protein.	Same as for B1, plus broccoli, skim milk, sweet potatoes and molasses
B6 (pyridoxine, pyridoxal, pyridoxamine, pyridoxamine-5-phosphate, pyridoxal-5-phosphate, alpha-pyracine, beta-pyracine	Protein, fat and carbohydrate metabolism, RNA, and DNA synthesis, antibody production, enzyme activator, hormone production (adrenalin and insulin) Uses include diabetes, kidney stones, arteriosclerosis, asthma, rheumatism, schizophrenia, nausea, vomiting, depression and menstruation symptoms.	Same as for B1, plus wheat germ and bananas
B12	Red blood cell formation, RNA and DNA synthesis, carbohydrate metabolism, healthy nervous system. Uses include pernicious anemia, and mental illnesses.	Same as for B1, plus salt water fish and oysters

Vitamin	Function & uses	Dietary sources
Biotin (vitamin H)	Protein, carbohydrate and unsaturated fatty acid metabolism. Deficiency causes hair loss and muscular pains.	Same as for B1, plus fish and wheat germ
C	Essential for good health, needed for healthy teeth, gums and tissues, builds strong body cells, fights virus infection, enhances iron absorption, essential for collagen formation. Prevents diabetes, bleeding gums, cholesterol build-up in blood vessels, atherosclerosis, common cold, lead, mercury and cadmium poisoning, recurrence of bladder and other forms of cancer and transformation of nitrites to toxic substances like nitrosamines. Antioxidant (keeps oxygen from forming toxic compounds).	Rose hips, citrus fruits, green peppers, broccoli, spinach, tomatoes, berries, cabbage, potatoes and green vegetables
D (sterols)	Essential for strong teeth and bones, calcium and phosphorus metabolism. Helps in regulating heart beat, prevents rickets and used in hypoparathyroidism.	Milk, egg yolk, livers and viscera of fish, cod liver oil, salmon and tuna
E (tocopherols)	Antioxidant, essential for red blood cells, dissolves fibrin, reduces thrombin formation and prevents fat absorption defects.	Wheat germ oil, vegetable oils, peanuts, green leafy vegetables, whole grains
Folic acid	Prevents anemia, certain mental disorders, controls cholesterol levels. Functions include red cell formation, maintenance of intestinal tract, and RNA and DNA synthesis.	Food yeast, meats, leafy green vegetables, endive, wheat bran, kale, spinach and turnips

Vitamin	Function & uses	Dietary sources
PABA (para-amino-benzoic acid)	Necessary for the synthesis of folic acid and utilization of pantothenic acid. Uses include certain rickettsial diseases, digestive and nervous disorders. Prevents sunburn and skin cancer.	Same as for B1
K	Blood clotting, synthesis of prothrombin by liver.	Green leafy vegetables, egg yolk, tomatoes, wheat germ, soybeans and potatoes
Inositol (meso-inositol)	Significance of this compound in human nutrition has not been established.	Fruits, meat, milk, nuts, vegetables, whole grains and yeast
Choline	Essential metabolite, synthesized in body, hence not a true vitamin. Essential ingredient of nerve fluid acetylcholine. Therapeutic applications include paralysis, cardiac arrest, kidney dysfunction, hypertension and nervous system function.	Brewer's yeast, fish, beef liver, soybeans and peanuts
P (bioflavonoids)	Effective substitute for hormone therapy, stops abnormal menstrual bleeding and capillary fragility, helps in hemorrhoids and varicose veins.	Lemon and other citrus fruits, vegetables and green peppers

Careful examination of Table 6.1 shows that all vitamins play an essential role in the proper functioning of various aspects of the human body. Single deficiencies are rare; usually multiple vitamin deficiencies are observed in many diseases.

A disease like diabetes, with its associated vascular complications, is a form of stress on the human body. Everyone knows what stress is, though a precise definition of the word is often difficult to achieve. The word stress, like success, failure or happiness, means different things to different people; except for a few specialized scientists, no one has really tried to define it although it has become a part of our daily vocabulary. Obviously, there are many different conditions in life that can produce stress: fatigue, pain, fear, humiliation, loss of blood and so on. Every one of these conditions can produce stress, and yet none of them can be singled out as being the only source of all stress. For our purposes, we would like to center on one very unique form of stress, namely, allergic reactions to specific foods and/or chemicals. In this sense, what we eat or the environment in which we live can and indeed does produce a form of biochemical stress that may result in a radical change of health. In order to determine whether or not allergic reactions to specific foods or chemicals were enough of a biochemical stress to alter the essential nutrient levels in susceptible individuals, we conducted an experiment on sixty-two patients with an average age of thirty-seven years. Forty-one of these patients were female; twenty-one were male. Although eighteen of these patients were diagnosed as schizophrenic, four as hyperactive, and one as an epileptic, all sixty-two manifested varying stages of the diabetic disease process.

The results of our experiment confirmed our suspicions: when each patient was tested for specific allergic responses that produced high blood sugar (diabetes), all sixty-two patients (i.e., 100 percent) registered significant utilization disorders of deficiencies in B6. Another very surprising and revealing fact was that 85 percent of them registered urine deficiencies in vitamin C. The precise clinical testing that was used to determine these results will be explained in detail later, but for now, the important point to realize is that maladaptively evoked produced high blood sugar reactions (diabetes) actually created deficiencies or utilization disorders of vitamin B6 and vitamin C in most of our patients. Moreover, 47 percent of our diabetic patients registered low in their test for folic acid. Other vitamin deficiencies were not measured, but there exists a probability of their related deficiencies.

What we observed in our clinic has some very interesting implications if seen in the light of scientific knowledge relating to nutrient deficiencies and arteriosclerosis. We observed, for example, that the stress of reactive foods (most commonly eaten foods to which patients become addicted), and other ecological factors including chemical addiction, can alter the susceptible person's body chemistry so much that deficiencies and abnormalities of certain essential nutrients occur. More specifically, this means that maladaptive food and chemical induced diabetic reactions set into motion a disturbed biochemical nutrient mechanism within the body that in turn can result in associated complications that are often as serious as the initial diabetic response. In order to see the significance of these clinically induced nutrient deficiencies, let us now turn our attention to an in-depth examination of some of the important scientific literature relating vitamin B6 deficiencies, vitamin C deficiencies, and folic acid deficiencies, as well as others, to the development of cardiovascular and cerebrovascular related diseases.

Studies indicate that there is indeed a relationship existing between diabetes and vitamin B6 deficiencies. When investigators at the Royal Perth Hospital in Australia took blood samples from more than five hundred diabetics, they found that vitamin B6 concentrations in these individuals were significantly lower than in healthy people. Moreover, those diabetics who were diagnosed as having cardiovascular problems had much lower levels of the vitamin than diabetics in general.[2] Similar results were achieved in the study of twenty-three diabetic patients at Japan's Wakayama Medical College Hospital. Dr. Yakito Kotake discovered that xanthurenic acid in a free form was invariably present in the urine of diabetic patients.[3] As far back as 1943, it was reported that the isolation of xanthurenic acid in the urine was an indication of a vitamin

B6 deficiency. Xanthurenic acid was then shown to be an abnormal metabolite of the amino acid tryptophan and was always related to a vitamin B6 deficiency. When vitamin B6 was added to the diet, xanthurenic acid immediately disappeared from the urine. Xanthurenic acid is formed and disappears almost universally under these conditions, and is excreted in the urine of rats, mice, dogs, pigs, monkeys and even humans whenever insufficient vitamin B6 is supplied.[4] As a result of this discovery, the trypto-phan loading test with its corresponding xanthurenic acid production was accepted as an accurate measurement of a B6 deficiency in human beings. It was precisely this test that was used in our clinic when allergic diabetic reac-tions were demonstrated to produce a vitamin B6 deficiency in 100 percent of our diabetic patients. Dr. Kotake also demonstrated by the use of the tryptophan loading test that his twenty-three diabetic patients had a vitamin B6 deficiency and/or utilization disorder.

Based on the preceding clinical evidence, we must concede that diabetic maladaptive reactions can actually produce a specific vitamin deficiency (in this case a vitamin B6 deficiency). But the question now arises as to precisely what consequences occur in the human body when a vitamin B6 deficiency is clinically recorded.

When protein is digested by the body, we have already seen that it is broken down into individual amino acids that compose it. One of these amino acids is named methionine. After several biochemical reactions, methionine is converted to homocysteine. Homocysteine is an extremely toxic chemical but, because it is regularly produced, the body quickly converts it to cystathionine. This is another chemical substance normally found in the body, but it is not toxic; in fact, it is entirely safe. In order to convert the toxic homocysteine chemical to a harmless cystathionine chemical, vitamin B6 is required. Patients with homo-cystinuria cannot convert homocysteine to cystathionine. As a result the former collects in the blood where it becomes a toxic substance. Since the conversion of homocysteine to cystathionine requires the presence of vitamin B6, this vitamin works much like a catalyst in this situation. If it is present in adequate amounts, the necessary chemical conversion works smoothly and rapidly. If, however, vitamin B6 is deficient or missing entirely, the production and abnormal build-up in the blood of homocysteine is the unhappy effect. As such, homocysteine is considered an abnormal metabolite of the essential sulphur containing amino acid methionine, much as xanthurenic acid is an abnormal metabolite of tryptophan.

When there are deposits of homocysteine in the blood or urine, we can accurately assume that there is a serious vitamin B6 deficiency. There are very dramatic biochemical consequences if and when this occurs. In 1969, Dr. Kilmer McCully of the Harvard Medical School and the Massachusetts General Hospital discovered that an elevated homocysteine concentration in the blood, produced by a vitamin B6 deficiency, could explain the initial vascular damage he discovered in the vitamin B6 deficient monkeys he was testing. As Dr. McCully technically explains: "The homocysteine effect of cellular proteoglycan synthesis is considered to be a key factor in the initiation of arteriosclerotic lesions because several lines of evidence from experimental and pathological literature show that changes in sulfate esterified proteoglycans are an essential feature of the evolution of the arteriosclerotic process."[5] Dr. McCully's technical explanation confirms our contention that elevated concentrations of homocysteine actually produce pathological changes in the arteries and other connective tissues. He concluded that in the absence of sufficient vitamin B6, homocysteine is inadequately converted to cystathionine. Homocysteine, therefore, will begin to collect in the blood and create abnormal metabolic pathways. These abnormal metabolic pathways eventually cause arteriosclerosis.

A study done in 1962 at the University of California School of Medicine in San Francisco by two brothers, Dr. Lewis Greenberg, professor of pathology, and Dr. David Greenberg, professor of biochemistry, further confirms the relationship existing between homocysteine, B6 deficiency, and the development of arteriosclerosis. Dr. Lewis Greenberg

speaks with authority about what he observed in arterial
changes when monkeys were fed vitamin B6 deficient
diets: "The monkeys were given a B6 deficient diet when
they were about one year old. They were fed this diet for a
year to a year and a half. From time to time we would have
to give them some B6 else they would have died. It is our
opinion that the longer the monkeys were on a vitamin B6
deficient diet, the more nearly their arteriosclerosis resem-
bled arteriosclerosis in human beings."[6] After critically
analyzing the monkeys' arteriosclerotic lesions caused by
the vitamin B6 deficiency, Dr. Greenberg said, "The monkeys' arteries showed a thickening of the intima (inner
lining of the artery), whereas the controlled monkeys (i.e.,
those monkeys given an adequate diet containing vitamin
B6) did not have this same thickening."[6] This particular
work with monkeys developing arteriosclerosis in relation
to vitamin B6 deficiency was repeated by Dr. C. W. Mushett
while working in the Merck Company Laboratories in the
United States.[7] In all clinically tested B6 deficient animals,
arteriosclerotic lesions were observed. The animals on the
vitamin B6 deficient diet for the longest periods had the
most widespread and advanced arteriosclerotic lesions. In
addition, coronary artery lesions were also noted in the
arteries of the kidney, and the pancreas. "There seems no
question," these scientists summarized their point, "that the
arterial lesions are related to pyridoxine (B6) deficiency.
The experimental lesions have a close resemblance to
arteriosclerosis as it occurs in man."[8]

More convincing evidence concerning the association
between a vitamin B6 deficiency and its relation to the
development of arteriosclerosis was offered by Dr. Nina
Carlson of Royal Belfast Hospital for Sick Children in
Northern Ireland. Dr. Carlson observed that some of the
retarded youngsters excreted homocysteine in their urine.
When the retarded children died at a very young age (i.e.,
seven to thirteen), autopsies revealed very advanced arteriosclerosis. Based on this study, and on all the other
previously mentioned studies, Dr. Carlson concluded that
the amino acid methionine needs vitamin B6 to complete its

metabolism in the human body. If there is an insufficient amount of vitamin B6 to do this job, homocystinuria (i.e., the development of homocysteine in the blood) will occur. The companions of homocystinuria are the vascular lesions that we associate with arteriosclerosis, the dreaded forerunner of heart disease.

The significant point about all the preceding clinical evidence is the fact that we now can assert that there truly is a causal biochemical link between diabetes and ateriosclerosis. We have seen, for example, that allergic addictive reactions can and do cause high blood sugar reactions. Associated with these high blood sugar reactions is a corresponding vitamin B6 deficiency. Once this vitamin is in low supply, clinical evidence suggests the development of homocystinuria; this particular biochemical disorder leads to arteriosclerosis. But the question now arises, what about our old friend cholesterol? Isn't the development of too much cholesterol in the blood the real problem underlying the progression of arteriosclerosis in diabetes? To answer this question, and in turn get a better insight into the relationship between cholesterol, vitamin B6, diabetes and arteriosclerosis, let us first define some terms.

Arteriosclerosis is the medical term describing hardening of the arteries. The most common form of this disease, the one that kills more Americans than any other disease, is atherosclerosis. The development of this disease follows this pattern: The inside walls of the arteries start deteriorating in their physical structure and small lesions begin to appear. This cellular deterioration of the inner walls of the arteries is fundamentally a result of a vitamin B6 deficiency. If the lesions become serious enough and if, as we shall see in a later chapter, there is an accompanying vitamin C deficiency (as is usually the case), capillary rupture and hemorrhaging (bleeding) begin to occur. The body then calls for a protective measure to stop the internal bleeding within the artery. This action is termed a blood clot (thrombosis), which seals off the hemorrhaging. At the site of the injury on the artery wall, dead and dying cells, white and red blood cells, continue to accumulate, and actually begin to occlude the artery. When this happens the blood supply is diminished, which in turn deprives the heart and the brain of life-giving blood.

As the injured area cells proliferate, they attract numerous substances, including calcium and cholesterol. While the calcium and cholesterol deposits continue to grow, they begin to form areas in the arteries called atheromos. The atheromos thicken and blood clots (thrombosis) begin to adhere, resulting in a severe reduction of blood circulation to the heart and to the rest of the body. As calcification continues, the arteries harden and high blood pressure ensues; circulation of the blood is then greatly diminished and a heart attack often results.

The important question that needs answering at this point in our discussion is whether our old TV villain, cholesterol, is the main causative factor in the development of arteriosclerosis and heart attacks, or whether it is merely an innocent bystander, like calcium, that gets caught up in a deterioration process of capillary rupture and lesions, hemorrhaging and blood clots, all of which are the body's response to the more underlying and fundamental causative factors of specific nutrient deficiencies. To answer this question more fully, let us now turn our attention to an in-depth examination of the function of cholesterol in the body.

Contrary to popular belief, physicians all know that cholesterol serves many important functions in the body, and is necessary for the optimum health of the whole person. Cholesterol found in the skin can be converted, for example, into vitamin D when exposed to sunlight or other ultraviolet light. Bile salts are derived from cholesterol. Cholesterol is involved with sex hormone production and with steroid hormone production by the adrenal gland, especially in times of severe stress. Cholesterol, therefore, is not a foreign or evil substance within the body. In fact, it is absolutely necessary for life!

Ever since the daily intake of dietary cholesterol was considered a major causative factor in coronary heart disease, the theory behind this type of thinking has had difficulties explaining serious inconsistencies. First of all, one of the inconsistencies is the fact that 80 percent of those who suffer heart attacks have normal cholesterol in their blood. Secondly, most of the cholesterol that exists in the body comes not from the dietary intake of fatty foods, but rather is produced by the body, and in particular by the liver. Blood levels of cholesterol do not correspond, therefore, to dietary levels of the substance in everyday situations. Of course, experimenters have induced heart disease by giving animals extremely large dosages of cholesterol. Clinical studies that have demonstrated such a relationship between cholesterol and the development of arteriosclerosis in animals must be seen, however, in the light of everyday human eating patterns. That is, in order for a high cholesterol diet to induce arteriosclerosis, as was done successfully in experimental animals, it must contain at least ten times the concentrations found in an ordinary human diet. Such a lopsided diet of intolerable amounts of fat would seem almost impossible to maintain for any length of time. Thus the findings that arteriosclerosis can be caused experimentally by a high dietary cholesterol intake may have little meaning for the human disease encountered in everyday life. Moreover, physicians at the Mayo Clinic have shown that the severity of arteriosclerosis is not always related to the levels of serum (blood) cholesterol, much less dietary cholesterol. They discovered, for example, that people with low serum cholesterol could have just as severe arteriosclerosis as those with high serum cholesterol.

Although the early work on the role of cholesterol in arteriosclerosis has been persuasive to some, especially TV advertisers of "low fat" products, there are other nagging discoveries that contradict our modern TV induced cholesterol mania. It has been discovered, for instance, that rabbits fed little or no cholesterol but large amounts of protein actually produced arterial lesions faster than rabbits fed diets high in cholesterol. Our discussion of methionine, homocysteine and vitamin B6 now reveals more clearly precisely why diets high in protein (and also high in methionine) and low in vitamin B6 can indeed produce serious arterial lesions. Furthermore, many experimental studies relating arteriosclerosis to high cholesterol are based on diets unknowingly high in methionine as well as cholesterol and other lipids. The question becomes whether the major villain in these studies is the cholesterol, or whether it is the homocysteine, producing arterial damage, which results in a cholesterol build-up at the damaged sites. It is our contention, based on empirical and clinical evidence, that the initial arterial damage of lesions, hemor- rhaging, blood clots and so on is first caused by specific nutritional deficiencies in the diet. Once the damaged area in the artery wall occurs, then the build-up of cholesterol as well as calcium becomes a secondary problem. But if one treats arteriosclerosis by simply reducing the dietary in- take of cholesterol, or for that matter calcium, one is merely treating the symptoms and not the cause of the disease. Cholesterol and calcium deposits should thus be seen as factors which follow the primary vascular damage caused by homocystinuria or vitamin B6 deficiency. As Roger Williams, Ph.D., of the Clayton Foundation, University of Texas at Austin, has stated: "It has come to be almost an orthodox position that if one wishes to protect against heart disease, one should avoid eating saturated fats. But the evidence shows that a high fat consumption, when accom- panied by plenty of the essential nutrients which all cells need, does not cause arteriosclerosis or heart disease. . . . For two hundred and eighty-five days rats were fed a diet containing 61.6 percent animal fat but highly superior in proteins, mineral and vitamin contents, without producing pathological changes in the aorta or in the heart. The animals did, to be sure, become obese, as much as three to four times their normal weight. There were no findings however, suggesting that either high animal fat diets or high vegetable fat diets were conducive under these conditions to arteriosclerosis." Obviously, a diet so rich in animal fat is not a healthy one. The problem of obesity adds to the risk of heart attack. We are, therefore, not advocating an extremely high fat diet. What is being said, however, is that the proper nutrient ratios (in this case vitamin B6) must always be maintained in any diet, whether it be low, moderate or high in fat, protein or carbohydrates. Further evidence that corroborates this type of thinking is suggested by the studies done of different dietary eating habits within various cultures throughout the world. Again, Dr. Roger Williams summarizes these results:

> In an extensive review of the various peoples of the earth who have little or no atherosclerosis and are virtually free of heart disease, Lowenstein found that the fat intake ranged from 21 grams per day to as much as 355 grams per day (Lowenstein, F.W., American Journal Clinical Nutrition, 15:175, 1964). In both the Somalis and the Samburus of East Africa, the diet is from 60 to 65 percent fat (animal), and yet they are nearly free from atherosclerosis and heart attacks. While it might be argued that ethnic differences are involved here, population groups of wide ethnic variation have been reported who subsist on high fat, high cholesterol, high caloric diets while remaining virtually free of coronary heart disease.

> In the text we have mentioned the report of Mann and his colleagues of the Masai tribe who subsist on a diet excessively high in butter fat (and cholesterol), the fat constituting as much as 60 percent of the total calories consumed, yet are virtually free of cardiovascular disease. Gsell and Mayer report that the isolated peoples of the Loetschental valley in the Valaisian Alps of Switzerland habitually eat a diet high in saturated fat and cholesterol, high in calories, but evidence low serum cholesterol values and little cardiovascular disorders (Gsell, D., and Mayer, J. "Low blood cholesterol associated with high calorie, high saturated fat intake in a Swiss Alpine village population." Am. J. Clin. Nutr., 1–:471, 1962).

> Stout and his co-workers report that an Italian immigrant colony in Roseta, Pennsylvania, consumes diets much richer in saturated animal fats than other Americans, yet [has] less than half the incidence of coronary heart disease (JAMA, 188:845, 1964).

> In a survey study of 27,000 Kenya East Indians, A.D. Charters and B. P. Arya report (Lancet, 1:288, 1960) that the animal fat consumption was relatively high among Punjabi non-vegetarian Gujeratis, but the percentage of heart disease

morbidity "is closely proportional to that of the population."
The statistics of their survey, conclude these investigators, suggest
that in the case of the East Indian population in Kenya, "the
ingestion of animal fats is not an important etiological factor" in
heart disease morbidity. Interestingly, besides their low animal
fat diet, the Gujerati vegetarians consume foods rich in polyunsaturated oils, as groundnut, cottonseed, and simsim oils, yet were
not "protected from coronary occlusion by a high intake of
unsaturated fatty acids."

In an epidemiological study of coronary heart disease in a
general population of 106,000 Americans conducted over a one
year period, W. J. Zukel and his co-workers found the highly
provocative fact that farmers showed a much lower incidence of
coronary heart disease than males of other groups, in spite of the
fact that there were no substantial differences in their mean
caloric intake or fat and cholesterol consumption (Zukel, W.J., et.
al., Am. J. Publ. Health, 49:1630, 1959).

In an epidemiological study of two Polynesian Island
groups, Hunter compared the diet, body build, blood pressure,
and serum cholesterol levels of the traditional-following Atiu
and Mitiaro with the more Europeanized Rarotongan neighbors
(Hunter, J.D., Fed. Proc., 21, Supp, 11:36, 1962). The Atiu-Mitiaro
people live on a diet low in calories and protein but rich in
highly saturated coconut fat. The Rarotongans eat more food, but
eat comparatively little coconut fat. Hunter found that 25
percent of the Rarotongans (males) suffered from hypertension as
compared to only 10 percent of the Atiu-Mitiaro males. While
the serum cholesterol levels of the saturated coconut fat-eating
Atiu-Mitiaro males were higher (as high as European males),
Hunter was unable to discover by electrocardiographic readings
any tendency to coronary heart disease.

Finally we turn to the early primitive Eskimo who subsisted
almost totally on an excessively high animal fat diet. In an early
1927 issue of the Journal of the American Medical Association
(May), in an article titled "Health of a Carnivorous Race," Dr.
William Thomas reports that of 142 adults between the ages of
forty and sixty who were completely examined, he found no
unusual signs of vascular or renal morbidity, and all indica-
tions were that diseases of the cardiovascular system were not
prevalent among these people. This is in agreement with other
reports of scientists of the primitive Eskimo (e.g., C. Lieb. JAMA,
July, 1926; V. Stefansson, in his book Cancer: Disease of

Civilization, p. 76; I.M. Rabinowitch, Canad. Med. Assoc. J., 31:487; W. Price, Nutrition and Physician Degeneration, New York: Hoeber, 1939).

It is clear, therefore, that adult males of widely differing ethnic stock can subsist on a high fat, high cholesterol, high caloric diet, and yet remain relatively free of cardiovascular disorders. Even if prevailing views are to the contrary, I think that the evidence points strongly toward the conclusion that the nutritional environment of the body cells—involving minerals, amino acids, and vitamins—is crucial, and that the amount of fat or cholesterol consumed is relatively inconsequential. . . .[9]

A large amount of information, based upon carefully controlled scientific experiments, indicates very strongly that vitamin B6 is another key nutrient which is often present in inadequate amounts in the cellular environment of those whose arteriosclerosis is extreme. Experiments with monkeys have yielded clear-cut results. When they are rendered vitamin B6 deficient, they develop arteriosclerosis rapidly. When monkeys are fed diets supplemented with vitamin B6, they have much lower levels of cholesterol in the blood than when these diets are not supplemented. The animals on the supplemented diet eat much more food than the others, and since their diet contains cholesterol, they get far more cholesterol into their bodies. This does not matter, however; the extra vitamin B6 they get allows them to dispose of the surplus, with the result that their cholesterol blood levels are not as high as in those animals that consume less cholesterol.[10]

The optimum intake of vitamin B6 thus affords a double benefit to those engaged in the battle against arteriosclerosis: It not only reduces their chances of developing homocysteine-induced arterial lesions, but it also reduces the serum cholesterol levels within their bodies. Knowing these facts, one becomes less and less impressed with the TV induced fad of cholesterol mania. The greatest proponent of reducing dietary cholesterol in the past has been the American Heart Association. Even they, however, have modified their previous position. Their new stance is an improvement, but they should also modify their public service advertisements to reduce cholesterol mania and the poor nutrition resulting from the public's fanaticism in its avoidance of nutrient rich foods containing cholesterol. As the American Heart Association states, "There is as yet no proof that a low cholesterol, low fat diet followed from early adult life will reduce the primary occurrence of heart attacks in Americans."[11]

We summarize this discussion by stating that dietary and/or plasma cholesterol levels by themselves are the major cause of arteriosclerosis. The problem occurs when the arterial walls begin to deteriorate and become clogged with dangerous metabolic debris (dead and dying cells, white and red blood cells, and so on) described earlier in this chapter. This process is, as we have seen, a result of specific nutrient deficiencies. At this time in the disease process, excessive amounts of plasma cholesterol become a very serious problem since they get caught up at the damaged arterial sites and thus further clog the arteries to a degree that often causes heart attacks and/or strokes. Knowing this, we must strive to eliminate all those dietary factors which cause the simultaneous occurrence of nutrient deficiencies as well as the excessive increase of blood cholesterol in the body. Let us now turn our attention to an examination of one such dietary factor.

There are many studies that indicate that dietary cholesterol, other things remaining equal, will have less of an effect on plasma (blood) cholesterol concentrations in humans than the effect of the quantity produced by the liver itself. These studies have demonstrated the fact that the major contributor to plasma cholesterol is in fact the liver.[12] Generally speaking, therefore, the concentrations of cholesterol in the blood appear to be determined largely by the amount synthesized by the liver. One dietary food substance that seems to accelerate the liver's synthesis of carbohydrates to fat (cholesterol) is the intake of table sugar (sucrose). Dr. P. T. Kuo, in a recent study at the University of Pennsylvania, found that dietary sugar administered to patients actually caused blood fats to increase.[13] In England, evidence has been presented by Dr. Yudkin and co-workers that excessive consumption of sugar is statistically associated with arteriosclerosis and heart attacks.[14]

Indeed, there are a growing number of studies[15] indicating that a high consumption of sugar is one of the factors causing the development of arteriosclerosis. Granted, this type of reasoning is completely contradictory to the old thinking that dietary cholesterol is the main factor causing arteriosclerosis. But let us consider this evidence: Our population's individual consumption of sugar has sky rocketed from ten pounds a year in 1910 to a frightening one hundred and twenty pounds per year in 1980. The consumption of such large amounts of sugar is an eating pattern of completely naked calories (i.e., no nutrients). As a result, this additional stress of consuming almost one-third of one's dietary caloric intake in sugar-coated, empty calories not only raises blood cholesterol, as the studies indicated, but it also sets the stage for conditions where vitamin B6 deficiencies (as well as other vitamin and mineral deficiencies) are more likely to occur.

Early in 1974, another experiment, this time in South Africa, also demonstrated the damaging effects of the consumption of too much refined carbohydrates. Thirty baboons (their physiology is similar to man's) were divided into five groups: There was one control group, fed nutrient rich foods, and there were four experimental groups which were fed a diet high in refined carbohydrates (sucrose, fructose, glucose, and bare starch). All four of the experimental groups developed varying degrees of substantial damage to their aortic arteries and had a 35 percent rise in blood cholesterol. But the group of baboons on the controlled diet consisting of whole wheat bread (high in vitamin B6), bananas (high in vitamin B6), yams, oranges (high in vitamin B6), carrots and so forth showed no damage to their aortas and no average rise in blood cholesterol. While this study only points a suggestive hand toward the fact that a diet high in strictly refined carbohydrates can cause serious arterial damage as well as an increased level of cholesterol in the blood, more studies should be done in this area. It does confirm our contention, however, that a diet high in refined carbohydrate foods (sucrose) actually deprives the body of the necessary nutrients required by our biochemistry for proper health and resistance to degenerative disease. As Dr. Yudkin points out: "A person assessed by our dietary history who is taking more than one hundred twenty grams of sugar a day (4 oz.) is perhaps five or more times as likely to develop myocardial infarction as one taking less than sixty grams a day."[16]

The contemporary American diet thus places a continuing strain upon metabolic processes. This diet is pernicious to the cardiovascular system not only because, as we have seen, continued addictive eating patterns create specific vitamin deficiencies which are in turn damaging to arterial integrity, but also because it tends to be quite high in empty calories, i.e., calories derived from highly processed refined carbohydrates, foods very rich in energy but low in the essential nutrients (e.g., vitamin B6, vitamin C and others) needed in the battle against arteriosclerosis. Hence, the American diet, despite its high caloric level, is not infrequently inadequate, relatively or absolutely, in specific vitamins needed to maintain healthy activity.

No one can state specifically how great each individual human's needs are for vitamin B6. It complicates the situation for some individuals' vitamin B6 requirements to be much higher than those of others who are on basically the same dietary eating pattern. And, of course, the requirement for vitamin B6 increases whenever there is an increased consumption of protein containing tryptophan and/or methionine, as well as an increased consumption of refined carbohydrates (sugar) and/or a very heavy consumption of fats. Such increased need levels for vitamin B6 are particularly distressing when seen in the light of some of the more recent studies done on the levels of vitamin B6 in foods found in America today. Henry Borsook of the California Institute of Technology, reviewing the amounts of B6 in diets, has reported that 20 to 30 percent of vitamin B6 is destroyed in vegetables when they are cooked. In the processing of wheat and white flour, 80 to 90 percent of the vitamin B6 is taken out with the bran, and the baking of it causes a 3.5 to 17.5 percent loss of this essential vitamin. He further quoted surveys that indicate a large proportion of American adults are not even receiving 1.5 mg of vitamin B6 daily.[17] Moreover, Wisconsin investigators found highly processed army K rations—a mixture of forty-five food items—inadequate with respect to vitamin B6 when fed to rats or to monkeys.[18] It has also been reported that heat sterilized milk, canned evaporated milk, or heat processed milk powders have a substantial amount of the vitamin B6 content destroyed, and that experimental rats cannot thrive on the milk treated in this way.[19]

In addition to these disturbing facts it is interesting to note that all pregnant women need even greater vitamin B6 supplements at the beginning of pregnancy and through-out its entire term. Moreover, since women need more vitamin B6 when estrogen is increased, as in the case of pregnancy, all women on estrogen birth control pills are also in need of more vitamin B6 daily. Out of an awareness of these statistics, John Ellis, M.D., states his case in the following manner: "In the light of these wide-spread deficiency conditions in this country, it is my opinion, as it is Paul Gyorgy's, that the minimum daily requirement for vitamin B6 should be changed from the present 2.5 mg daily to 25 mg a day. There also should be 100 mg of vitamin B6 in every prenatal capsule and 50 mg in each supplementary vitamin tablet for therapeutic use. It is also my conviction, after eleven years of clinical studies with vitamin B6, that the minimum daily requirement for all infants and children under twelve years of age should be set at 10 mg. When these concepts are accepted, in my opinion, a lot of disease is going to disappear in this civilized world. I have seen enough husbands and wives who ate from the same table and who suffered from the same symptomology to conclude positively that vitamin B6 deficiency is the most prevalent deficiency disease in the United States today."[20]

If you have any doubts about the validity of Dr. Ellis's statement that vitamin B6 deficiency is the most prevalent deficiency disease in the United States today, consider the following example. In a study of forty-six thousand women, half were taking birth control pills and half were not. Both groups were equivalent in age and marital status. For the young women who had taken the pill continuously for five years or more, vascular disease leading to death was ten times greater than that of the controlled group. As we have seen, the homocysteine theory holds that a reduced vitamin B6 level, attributable in this case to taking the estrogen pill, causes an increase in the toxic level of homocysteine in the blood. This of course leads to further cardiovascular degeneration. Indeed, the problem is real, and necessitates further research.

In this chapter we have centered our attention on one specific nutrient, i.e., vitamin B6. Nothing we have said about this specific nutrient deficiency should obscure the fact that diabetes, and its related cardiovascular diseases, will have their roots in a number of nutritional deficiencies. For example, studies have clearly indicated that a vitamin B1 deficiency (beri-beri), if prolonged, seriously damages the heart.[21] In fact, no essential mineral, amino acid or vitamin can safely be excluded from consideration in connection with heart disease.[22] But before we continue with our studies of other nutrients and their relationship to arteriosclerosis, let us summarize by saying that the clinical data previously mentioned highlights the proposition that, as Roger Williams states, "High or low amounts of fats or carbohydrates are not atherogenic providing supportive nutrients, specifically pyridoxine (vitamin B6), are present. But if pyridoxine is not adequately provided, regardless of the relative amounts of fat or carbohydrate, the diet will be atherogenic."[23] Thus, instead of counting calories, or worrying about the relative amounts of fats, proteins or carbohydrates that are in the diet, one should rather center one's attention on the *nutrient ratios* in reference to the amount of general food categories. For as we have seen, if the nutrient ratios of vitamin B6 are adequate, the fat, carbohydrate and protein will handle themselves, and no arteriosclerosis will likely develop.

Parenthetically speaking, an interesting new research area with which we recently became involved is the relationship existing between total vitamin B6 metabolism and methionine metabolism. Cystine is a necessary amino acid which the body makes from the essential amino acid methionine. The metabolic steps for this conversion are: methionine to cystathionine (a previously mentioned metabolic process requiring vitamin B6), cystathionine to cysteine, and finally, cysteine to cystine. What is particularly interesting here is the fact that while looking for multifactor biochemical abnormalities in our diabetic patients and other patients with chronic degenerative diseases, we discovered a startling connection between these diseases and the conversion process of vitamin B6. We observed that most of our patients lacked the capability of converting vitamin B6 into the active coenzyme form, pyridoxal-5-phosphate. We believe that the culprit in this vitamin B6 conversion problem is the amino acid cystine. Just as vitamin B6 is needed for the proper conversion of methionine to cystathionine, so too is the end product of this biochemical chain (cystine) needed for the breakdown and utilization by the body of vitamin B6 into pyridoxal-5-phosphate. The interdependency and/or interrelatedness of these chemicals is thus established as an important biochemical mandate for the proper functioning of the human body.

What is even more significant here is the fact that any blocking of methionine metabolism prior to the formation of cystine will have the consequence of increasing S-adenosyl methionine, which in turn will produce an excessive production of methionine enkephalin. This last chemical has an addictive morphine-like activity in the body that is equal to a hundred times the potency of morphine. Consequently, with any form of food and/or chemical addiction that establishes a vitamin B6 and methionine metabolism disorder, the body actually evokes its own addictive chemical narcotics (e.g., methionine enkephalin) out of this disordered metabolism. There are, of course, other disordered amino acid metabolisms that produce similar narcotic-like chemicals. All these self-produced chemical narcotics are as equally addicting—and in some cases more so—as any externally supplied narcotics such as morphine or heroin. The body thus reinforces, unfortunately, food and chemical addiction by producing narcotic-like chemicals within itself that act in such a way as to further enslave the addict in his or her own habituating activities.

We believe that these new findings provide for an entirely new outlook and understanding concerning the chronic degenerative disease process. No more can we be satisfied with giving one essential nutrient with the expectations of miraculous cures. The teamwork principle (Williams) of nutrients working together toward a healthy biochemical functioning within the body must always be honored when treating a patient from an Orthomolecular-Ecologic point of view. With some patients it is better to give vitamin B6 alone. Others require cystine and vitamin B6, while still others do better on cystine and pyridoxal-5-phosphate. These differences are all determined by the patient's unique biochemical individuality and must be tested and treated accordingly. The future of Orthomolecular-Ecologic Medicine will lie in all the exciting discoveries concerning the countless numbers of biochemical interactions existing among the various amino acids, vitamins, minerals, trace elements, hormones and enzymes in the body. Let us, therefore, turn our attention to other nutrients significantly involved in the disease of diabetes and arteriosclerosis.

REFERENCES

1. Lowenstein, B. E. 1976. *Diabetes*. New York; Harper and Row, p. 227.

2. Australian and New Zealand Journal of Medicine (Dec. 1977).

3. Kotake, Y. 1957. Experiments of chronic diabetic symptoms caused by xanthurenic acid. *Clinical Chemistry* 3:432–436.

4. Lepkovsky, S., et al. 1943. *Journal of Biological Chemistry* 149:195; Miller, E. C. 1945. *Journal of Biological Chemistry* 157:551; Cartwright, G. E. 1944. *Bulletin, Johns Hopkins Hospital* 75:35; Greenberg, L. D. 1948. *Federation Proceedings* 7:157.

5. McCully, K. S. 1970. Importance of homocysteine-induced

abnormalities of proteoglycan structure of arteriosclerosis. *American Journal of Pathology.* 59 (1):181–193.

6. Mushett, C. W. March 1956. Arteriosclerosis in pyridoxine-deficient monkeys and dogs. *Federation Proceedings* 15:526; Rinehart, J. F. 1949. Arteriosclerotic lesions in pyridoxine-deficient monkeys. *American Journal of Pathology* 25:481–491; McCully, K. S. July 1969. Vascular Pathology of homocysteinemia: implications for the pathogenesis of arteriosclerosis. *American Journal of Pathology* 56:111–128.

7. Mushett, C. W. Arteriosclerosis in pyridoxine-deficient monkeys and dogs, p. 526.

8. Gibson, J. B. July 1964. Pathological findings in homocystinuria. *Journal of Clinical Pathology* (17(4):427–437.

9. Williams, R. J. 1973. *Nutrition Against Disease.* New York: Bantam Books, p. 249.

10. *Ibid.* 252–253.

11. American Heart Association. 1972. *Clinical Chemistry.*

12. Eckles, N. E., et al. 1955. *Journal of Laboratory and Clinical Medicine* 46:359; Tennent, D. 1957. *Journal of Biological Chemistry* 228:241; Triedman, M., et al. 1951. *American Journal of Physiology* 164:789.

13. Kuo, P. T., et al. 1967. Dietary carbohydrates in hyperlipemia. *Journal of Clinical Nutrition* 20:116.

14. Yudkin, J. 1957. Diet and coronary thrombosis. *Lancet* 2:155.

15. Kaufman, N. A. 1966. Changes in the serum lipid levels of hyperlipemic patients following the feeding of starch, sucrose, and glucose. *American Journal of Clinical Nutrition* 18:261; Kuo, P. T. 1965. *Clinical Investment* 44:1924; Antar, M. A. 1963. *Federation Proceedings* 22:327.

16. Yudkin, J. 1964. Dietary fat and dietary sugar in relation to ischemic heart disease and diabetes. *Lancet* 2:4.

17. Borsook, Henry. 1964. The relation of the vitamin B6 human requirement to the amount in the diet. *Vitamins and Hormones* 22:855–874.

18. Tappan, D. V. 1953. Observation on the nutrition of rhesus monkeys receiving highly processed rations. *Journal of Nutrition* 51:469.

19. Tomarelli, R. M. 1955. Biological availability of vitamin B6 of heated milk. *Journal of Agricultural Food Chemistry* 3:338.

20. Ellis, J. M. 1973. *Vitamin B6: The Doctor's Report.* New York: Harper and Row, pp. 207–208.

21. Wintrobe, M. M. 1943. Electrocardiographic changes associated with thiamine deficiency in pigs. *Bulletin, Johns Hopkins Hospital* 73:169; Ashburn, L. L. 1944. Development of cardiac lesion in the thiamine-deficient rats. *Archives of Pathology* 37:27; Swank, R. L. 1941. The production and study of cardiac failure in thiamine-deficient dogs. *American Heart Journal* 22:154.

22. Follis. 1956. The effects of nutritional deficiency on the heart: a review. *American Journal of Clinical Nutrition* 4:107.

23. Williams, R. J. 1971. *Nutrition Against Disease*, p. 246.

CHAPTER SEVEN

Vitamin C against degenerative and infectious diseases

As far back as 1934, Dr. C. G. King of the University of Pittsburgh demonstrated that guinea pigs maintained on very low levels of vitamin C developed degeneration of the islets of Langerhans located in the pancreas.[1] This particular area of the pancreas, of course, is that section within the gland that produces insulin. In addition, these vitamin C deficient guinea pigs demonstrated an extremely low sugar tolerance level, which was rapidly regained upon feeding them high levels of vitamin C. Dr. King's initial study was proven to be correct by a more comprehensive series of experimental tests done in India by Dr. S. Banerjee in 1943.[2] Dr. Banerjee not only demonstrated that guinea pigs with scurvy (extreme vitamin C deficiency) manifested poor sugar tolerance, but he also showed that the pancreas's production in the vitamin C deficient pigs was reduced to about one-eighth that of normal guinea pigs. In addition, he observed gross changes in the microscopic appearance of the pancreas in the vitamin C deficient guinea pigs. This abnormal appearance returned to normal when the guinea pigs were given vitamin C. Based on the evidence discovered in this study he made the following conclusions: "The disturbed carbohydrate metabolism as seen in scurvy is due to a deficiency of insulin secretion, and a chronic deficiency of vitamin C may be one of the etiological factors (causes) of diabetes mellitus in human subjects."[3]

Other studies have given similar results with guinea pigs deprived of vitamin C. Altenburger demonstrated that guinea pigs deprived of vitamin C were unable to convert glucose to glycogen for storage in their livers. As a result, a dose of insulin that produced a pronounced decline in blood sugar in normal monkeys had little effect on monkeys deficient in vitamin C.[4] In the light of this study, as well as all other experimental evidence, it is safe to conclude that there does indeed exist a clear relationship between a disturbed insulin and glucose metabolism and a vitamin C deficiency. This relationship is seen not only in experimental animals that have scurvy, but in other animals maintained on a diet deficient in vitamin C.

If we look at the partnership existing between vitamin C and insulin from another point of view, it has been observed that vitamin C potentiates the action of insulin. This is to say that vitamin C makes it possible to derive the same desired biochemical effect with much less insulin. Dr. J. Frederick Dice of Stanford University, for example, had been diagnosed as a juvenile diabetic at the age of fifteen and required thirty-two units of insulin daily. During an experiment, which lasted twenty-three days, this dosage was gradually reduced by him to thirteen units a day. The reason for this reduction of insulin was his hourly ingestion of vitamin C from 7 A.M. to 12 midnight. The interesting point here is that megadoses of vitamin C may make it possible for the diabetic patient to reduce drastically his or her insulin requirements.[5] Other studies by Rogoff[6] and Pfleger[7] also imply that high levels of vitamin C can improve the action of insulin in diabetic patients. The patients in these studies actually controlled their sugar carbohydrate metabolism with lower levels of insulin by ingesting large dosages of vitamin C.

Above and beyond the previously mentioned uses of vitamin C, Bio-Ecologic physicians are finding that megadoses of vitamin C can be used to prevent or delay the vascular complications of diabetes. The rationale for this type of therapy is offered by Dr. George B. Mann of Vanderbilt University.[8] Dr. Mann originally thought that insulin was required for the transport of vitamin C into the cells of certain tissues. Recently he experimentally discovered that impaired insulin function does indeed inhibit the transport of vitamin C to essential tissues, resulting in a kind of "local tissue scurvy" within the body. Couple this discovery with our knowledge that animals maintained on low levels of vitamin C actually develop degeneration of the insulin producing islets of Langerhans and you have a biochemically explosive situation in which deficiencies of vitamin C levels in the body cause lower levels of insulin production, while at the same time these low levels of insulin further complicate and inhibit the proper transport of vitamin C to important tissues throughout the body.

To indicate the sort of phenomena Dr. Mann has in mind when he refers to "local tissue scurvy," let us examine some more facts about vitamin C and its relation to strong healthy arteries. One of the most essential biochemical functions of vitamin C in our body is the formation, synthesis and maintenance of a protein-like substance called collagen. It cannot be formed without the presence of vitamin C. Collagen, which is the body's most important structural substance, can be likened to a ground substance or cement base that supports and holds the tissues and organs together. Without it in the body, all of us would literally dissolve away into nothingness. It is responsible for over one-third of our body's total weight and, as such, is the most extensive tissue system.

In relation to diabetes, we know that collagen strengthens and supports the structures of arteries and veins, being like a tissue cement within these structures; if there is a

deficiency in the structure of collagen, then our arteries
rupture and bleed. As Irwin Stone suggests:

> As early as 1941, it was suspected that an inadequate intake
> of ascorbic acid was a factor in coronary thrombosis due to
> impaired collagen production, causing capillary rupture and
> hemorrhage in the arterial walls. Blood plasma, ascorbic acid
> measurements were made in four hundred and fifty-five consecu-
> tive adult patients admitted to the Ottawa Civic Hospital over a
> seven month period, and it was found that fifty-six percent had
> sub-normal levels (below 0.5 mg percent) and eighty-one percent
> of the coronary patients were in the sub-normal range. It was
> recommended that patients with coronary artery disease be
> assured of an adequate vitamin C (ascorbic acid) intake. A 1947
> paper showed that inadequate ascorbic acid body levels were
> not limited to cardiac patients of the lower economic brackets.
> The survey included five hundred and fifty-six private patients,
> of which one hundred and twenty-three had organic heart disease.
> Forty-two percent of all patients, fifty-nine percent of the heart
> patients, and seventy percent of the coronary thrombotic patients
> had low plasma levels of ascorbic acid (below 0.5 mg percent).
> Sixty-five percent of the coronary group had dangerously low
> levels (0.35 mg percent or less). Again it was suggested that
> ascorbic acid be used as an adjunct to the usual methods of
> treatment, especially in the long range care in the postinfarctive
> period.[9]

The end result of vitamin C deficiency is thus "local
tissue scurvy," or the thickening of vascular basement
membranes, fragility of blood vessel walls throughout the
entire body, as well as hemorrhaging within the vessel
walls. When such damage is done to the vessel walls
within the heart, it is called a miocardio-infarction; when it
happens in the eyes, it is called retinopathy; and when it
happens in the kidneys, it is called nephropathy. Diabetics,
however, as Dr. Mann admonishes, may not show the
more general signs of classic scurvy because their vitamin C
intake may be sufficient to reach tissues that are not
insulin sensitive, yet insufficient for those (as previously
mentioned) that are.

A protective measure called a blood clot (thrombosis)
usually occurs in "local tissue scurvy," since the artery

wall has been injured and is bleeding. "Thrombosis," writes McCormick, "is not in itself a pernicious development but rather a protective response of the organism designed normally to effect repair of damaged blood vessels. High blood pressure, excessive stretching of blood vessels and deficiency of vitamin C (ascorbic acid), resulting in rupture and bleeding of the intima at the site of such stress, initiate the development of the thrombosis by means of the clotting of the blood, which is also a protective reaction. This multiple protective mechanism should be sustained and controlled by physiological means (vitamin C therapy) rather than suppressed by anti-coagulants with their dangerous side effects."[10]

In addition to the studies showing how arterial wall damage occurs with a vitamin C deficiency, Dr. Roger Williams has cogently argued that this specific nutrient is also related—when not supplied in optimum amounts—to the development of arterial lesions, much as in the case of vitamin B6 deficiency. As Dr. Williams states, "Willis demonstrated that an ascorbic acid deficiency in the guinea pigs resulted in 'arterial lesions morphologically typical of atherosclerosis' (Canadian Medical Association Journal, 69:17, 1953). Ascorbic acid injections into guinea pigs with cholesterol-fed induced atherosclerosis had a marked effect inhibiting the atherosclerotic conditions. . . . In 1955 Willis also discovered that a localized ascorbic acid depletion often existed in segments of arteries afflicted with atherosclerosis. Adjacent arterial segments without lesions had a higher ascorbic acid content, and atherosclerosis was rare in these arteries (Canadian Medical Association Journal, 72:500, 1955)."[11]

The implications of Dr. Williams's thinking are deadly: when you find a significant level of bleeding and fragility in the artery wall, coupled with lesions caused by a vitamin C and a vitamin B6 deficiency, you have a perfect site in the damaged artery for cholesterol and calcium deposits to collect. Once this occurs, of course, the blood flow within the artery is diminished, and the death-dealing effects of this process quickly ensue. To add fuel to this already serious biochemical fire, researchers[12] have discovered that the greater the deprivation of vitamin C, the more the cholesterol accumulates in our bodies. Similarly, other studies[13] have clearly demonstrated that the intake of high levels of vitamin C actually brings down cholesterol levels in rabbits, guinea pigs, rats and in humans.

All of these provocative research studies conducted around the world for the last four decades strongly suggest that the ingestion of optimum levels of vitamin C and vitamin B6, as well as other nutrients, should be implemented as a prophylactic regime to prevent the high incidence of arteriosclerosis and other cardiovascular complications so associated with diabetes. If such a specific Bio-Ecologic treatment program is practiced clinically, we assert that these optimal levels of both vitamin B6 and vitamin C—and other nutrients of course—will indeed offer the best means of effecting a prophylactic measure against the development of arterial lesions, initial arterial hemorrhaging with its associated thrombosis, as well as a perfectly safe means by which to maintain healthy levels of cholesterol in the body.

But what is most important is the fact that our clinical evidence with diabetics empirically confirms the need for this type of treatment: 100 percent of our patients manifested deficiency in vitamin B6 and a corresponding 85 percent of them showed a deficiency in vitamin C. We believe, therefore, that the associated arterial complications in these diabetic patients are explainable functions of a variety of specific nutrient deficiencies (i.e., vitamin C, vitamin B6, and so on). These deficiencies are initially caused by the disease process of allergy-addiction. But please bear in mind that if there are adequate levels of vitamin C and vitamin B6, as well as other nutrients, and if all food and chemical allergies are eliminated, then the arterial damage associated with these nutrient deficiencies and allergy addictions is not likely to occur. The additional bonus of specific nutrients lowering cholesterol levels further aids in our protection against the cardiovascular complications of diabetes.

The role of infection

Microorganisms (i.e., bacteria, fungi, viruses) are as much a part of the environment as foods, chemicals and inhalants. Figuratively speaking, they are constantly trying to "eat us alive." Sometimes they succeed! If we die of other causes, they eventually eat the physical remains. Only healthy cells, tissues and organs within our bodies can effectively defend against these numerous environmental microorganisms. Whenever there is any form of allergic reaction to food and/or chemicals or inhalants that compromises the homeostatic state of our cells, tissues and organs, these microorganisms take over by invasion, multiplication and production of toxins. The diabetic disease process is well documented as decreasing the immunologic defense against such a microorganism invasion. For example, it has been known for years that diabetics have more infections than do nondiabetics. "Now it has been shown," writes Leo Krall, "that the natural body defense against infection may be defective in poorly regulated diabetes. Phagocytes [the white cells that help to fight infection] appear to be much less effective in uncontrolled diabetes."[14]

In addition to being an effective weapon used in the battle against the cardiovascular complications of diabetes, vitamin C is also a potent agent that can be used in conquering all the different forms of infectious diseases. Let us now, therefore, examine precisely how this vitamin is used by several Bio-Ecologic physicians in the continuing struggle with infectious diseases.

Bio-Ecologic Medicine aims primarily at the achievement and preservation of optimum health and the prevention and treatment of disease by regulating the concentration of chemical molecules normally present in the human body. One of these molecules important in the treatment of infectious disease is vitamin C. To appreciate why optimum daily intake of this nutrient is so essential in the battle against infectious disease, we must first remember that man has a genetic defect that prevents him from making his own supply of vitamin C inside his body. This is not true for most other animals. They manufacture ascorbic acid (vitamin C) either in their kidneys or in their livers, and thus do not need an external source for this necessary nutrient. The mammals that have been clinically examined in this respect range from a mouse, weighing less than one ounce, to a goat, weighing about seventy-five pounds, and the amounts of vitamin C manufactured by these two animals are approximately proportionate to their body weights. The mouse, for example, is reported to make the equivalent of 19 grams per day, calculated on the basis of 70 kilograms body weight, and the goat 13 grams per day, measured on the same basis. These normal daily levels increase dramatically when the animal is placed under a stress situation such as an infectious flareup. Our experience is that nature's workings are in the main reliable, so it would seem safe to assume that it is unlikely that these animals would synthesize more ascorbic acid than needed for optimum health. But the controversial question now arises as to what amounts of this particular vitamin are needed to put a man, who does not manufacture his own vitamin C, in the best of health and give him the greatest immunological protection against infectious diseases of all kinds.

In order to answer this, we must first understand the concept of RDA—Recommended Dietary Allowance—as formulated by the Food and Nutrition Board of the National Academy of Sciences, National Research Council. Most lay people interpret RDA for any particular nutrient—in this case vitamin C—as being the specific dosage that leads to the best of health for all people. That is, if I take the RDA of vitamin C every day of my life, I will more than likely achieve the best of health that can possibly be gained by the intake of this nutrient. This interpretation is quite false. The truth of the matter is that the RDA is only the estimated amount that, for most people, will prevent scurvy or death caused by overt vitamin deficiency. It does not take into account biochemical individuality, i.e., individual levels of nutrients needed for optimum health. This point is very important and should be understood thoroughly. Dr. Harper, the chairman of the Committee on Recommended Dietary Allowances of the Food and Nutrition Board, has clearly stated that the RDAs "are not recommendations for the ideal diet." "They were adopted," added Dr. Hegsted, another nutritionist, "to avoid any implication of finality or optimal requirements."[15] In short, the Board's recommendations were adopted so as to indicate to the general public those amounts of vitamin C needed in order to avoid scurvy. The same is true, of course, for all the other nutrients and their related deficiency diseases.

The problem with the Board's recommendations is that the medical profession took hold of them and created a misconception now generally accepted by many physicians. This misconception is based on the following reasoning: Lack of ascorbic acid causes scurvy. If there are no signs or symptoms of scurvy, we must assume that there is no deficiency whatever of ascorbic acid. Therefore, there is no need to take supplements of this vitamin. The first sentence of this three part deduction is a medical fact. However, the problem arises with the false assumption that, since there are no symptoms of scurvy, there is absolutely no need for any additional intake of vitamin C. You see, scurvy is not just a symptom of a deficiency, but a final collapse, a death syndrome manifesting itself in a total breakdown and disintegration of our biochemical being. But there is a very large gray area—i.e., colds, infections, flu, degenerative disease—existing between the total blackness of scurvy and death and the pure white of optimum health and resistance to disease. And it is precisely in this gray area, so to speak, that we must answer the important question: what intake of vitamin C is needed by man in order to achieve optimum health and resistance to disease rather than barely avoid developing scurvy? No longer can we be satisfied with the misconception that if we do not have scurvy, we do not need any additional amounts of vitamin C in order to achieve the optimum health possible for our particular biochemical being. And no longer can we be satisfied with the uninformed opinion that the RDA alone will guarantee our optimum health. At this point, what we can be guaranteed is that if we do take the RDA of vitamin C, we will very likely not develop scurvy. The question still remains, however: What if a man takes greater amounts of vitamin C than the RDA? Will these greater concentrations of this particular nutrient increase his resistance to infections and/or degenerative disease and thereby give him better health than if he had not taken them?

According to Dr. Linus Pauling, "There is overwhelming clinical evidence that an increased intake of vitamin C, that is, several times the RDA of 45 mg per day for an adult, provides significant protection against the common cold."[16] Several double-blind scientific studies conducted over a span of years ranging from 1942 to 1975 all confirm Pauling's thinking that an increased intake of ascorbic acid (and other nutrients, of course) strengthens man's natural protective mechanisms of the body, and thus decreases both the number of colds and the severity of individual colds. The results of these double-blind studies are as follows:[17]

	(Reduction in illness)
Cowan, Diehl, Baker: Minnesota, 1942	31 percent
Ritzer: Switzerland, 1961	63 percent
Charleston, Clegg: Scotland, 1972	58 percent
Anderson, Reid, Beaton: Canada, 1973	32 percent
Coulehan, Reisinger, Rogers, Bradley: Arizona, 1974	30 percent
Sabiston, Radonski: Canada, 1974	68 percent
Anderson, Beaton, Corey, Spero: Canada, 1975	25 percent
Average reduction in illness due to an increased intake of vitamin C:	44 percent

The amounts of ascorbic acid taken in these preceding double-blind studies varied from 200 mg to 2000 mg (2 grams). These positive results were achieved because of the functions that vitamin C performs in the body. Let us, therefore, examine these functions.

Probably the most important and potent defense mechanism that the body has is the total destruction of invading opportunist and infectious microorganisms by the leukocytes or white blood cells of the blood. This process is called phagocytosis. It was clinically established as long as thirty years ago that vitamin C is one of the most important ingredients for the proper and effective phagocytic activity of man's leukocytes. Indeed, leukocytes can only maintain their phagocytic activity against infectious microorganisms, engulfing them and destroying them, if the leukocytes contain optimum levels of vitamin C; that is, unless the white blood cells are totally saturated with ascorbic acid, they are like soldiers without bullets. The white blood cells have the ability to ingest the bacterial microorganisms, and when they do, they simultaneously produce hydrogen peroxide. This chemical then must combine with vitamin C to produce a substance that is lethal to almost all known bacteria. If the proper levels of vitamin C are not present at the biochemical war site, the white blood cells' battle against the microorganisms will be lost. Drs. Hume and Weyers in Scotland[18] reported in 1973 that an ordinary diet usually does not contain adequate amounts of vitamin C needed for proper phagocytic action of the white blood cells during the stress situation of a cold. Even an intake of two hundred and fifty milligrams a day is not enough to maintain phagocytically effective amounts. Normally, however, an intake of one to fifteen grams daily during an infectious stress situation like a cold is enough concentration to enable this natural mechanism of protection against bacterial disease to operate. But even these large amounts are sometimes not enough, depending on the specific infectious microorganisms involved.

Many scientists, physicians and nutritionists have reported that vitamin C in large dosages inactivates all forms of viruses *in vitro*. Technically speaking, Murata and Kitagawa believe that this inactivation results from the splitting of the nucleic acid of the virus by free radicals formed during the oxidation of vitamin C. Viruses of poliomyelitis, vaccina, hoof-and-mouth, rabies, hepatitis, pneumonia, measles, chicken pox, mononucleosis, encephalitis and others have all been destroyed in experiments by the optimum dosages of ascorbic acid. When attempting to treat any of the preceding infections with vitamin C, individual optimum dosages of the nutrient are best determined by adopting Dr. Robert F. Cathcart's principle of "bowel tolerance level." He explains this concept in the following way:

About seven years ago I began to hear rumors about Dr. Pauling saying something about vitamin C and the common cold. I had been a person who had suffered all my life with hay fever, having had injections since the age of nine. I was also one of those persons who had colds all the time. So I started taking vitamin C and found that I could give up my injections for hay fever, and also that my colds were under control. But then I went on and discovered something very interesting: I was able to take an amount of vitamin C when I was ill with a cold that I couldn't possibly tolerate when I was well. We elaborated on that a little bit and started experimenting with patients. After clinical testing, we came up with what I call bowel tolerance concept in determining the dose of vitamin C that should be given patients. . . . Bowel tolerance levels of vitamin C means you let the body take as much vitamin C as it needs until diarrhea occurs. Once you get diarrhea, you cut back a couple or more grams until the diarrhea goes away. This practice lets the body use that amount of vitamin C proportional to the amount of toxin that is around. . . . The astonishing thing about bowel tolerance levels of vitamin C is that the same person—the patient who when well gets diarrhea on say 12 grams—when ill with a moderate cold can take 30 to 60 grams without diarrhea; with a bad cold or flu, 100–150 grams, and with viral diseases such as mononucleosis or viral pneumonia, I have used in excess of 200 grams a day without producing diarrhea. In some cases the body evidently needs that much, albeit for only a short time. . . . Essentially, the sicker you are, the more you can take, and taking enough—and that is important—seems to detoxify you. You get well quickly! As you do, you will find that you can tolerate less and less ascorbic acid until you go back to normal when you are well. Remember, everyone else has been talking about a fixed dose of vitamin C. Those studies go from two to maybe four grams a day, and they sometimes see little chemical or statistical effect. That doesn't surprise me. If you have a 100 gram flu bug—it's my custom to put a number before the name of the disease to represent the amount of vitamin C that the patient can consume the first couple of days of the disease without diarrhea—and thus take roughly 100 grams of vitamin C, you will quickly eliminate 90 percent of the symptoms of the disease. But if you treat a 100 gram bowel tolerance level flu bug with 2 or even 20 grams a day, you will not see much happen.[19]

The following graph represents Dr. Cathcart's clinical findings concerning average minimum dosages of vitamin C per twenty-four hours needed to neutralize acute symptoms of disease.

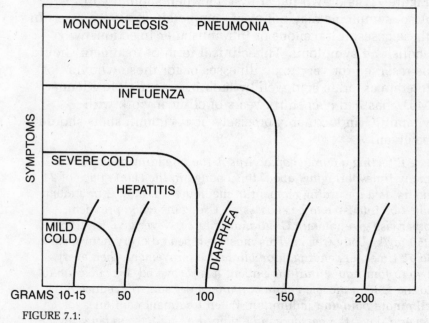

FIGURE 7.1:

Dr. Cathcart's Minimum Dose of Vitamin C per 24 Hours to Neutralize Acute Symptoms of Disease

Note that the amount of vitamin C necessary to produce diarrhea in Figure 7.1 increases more or less proportionately to the toxicity of the disease. Bowel tolerance levels of vitamin C are obviously greater for pneumonia than they are for a severe cold. Also, these levels increase somewhat according to the degree of other stress related factors: allergy addiction, maladaptive reactions, heat, cold, anxiety, drinking, cancer, injury, surgery, psychosis, arthritis and so forth. It is important to understand that 80 percent of the population tolerates half a gram to ten grams of ascorbic acid when well; most of the remainder get diarrhea somewhere in these levels. However, when those who tolerate it poorly are sick their tolerance approaches the levels of the other 80 percent.

Acute symptoms are affected very little until 90 percent of the bowel tolerance is reached. Then the symptoms drop off suddenly. This is the reason the symptom curve in Figure 7.1 is drawn flat at first and then suddenly drops. Also, symptoms may not clear completely in severe cases. In these cases, intravenous or intramuscular injections will abolish all symptoms. This clinical form of treatment should be reserved for very toxic illnesses or for those who do not tolerate ascorbic acid well by mouth. Frederick R. Klenner, M.D., has had over thirty years of clinical work with vitamin C and explains precisely how vitamin shots should be given:

Effecting a cure when a virus is the offending agent, and many times [bringing] about this change in the short space of 24 hours, is a rewarding moment in medicine. Vitamin C treatment must be intensive to be successful. Use veins when practical, otherwise give vitamin C intramuscularly. Never give less than 350 mg/kg body weight. This must be repeated every hour for up to 12 times, depending upon clinical improvement, then every two to four hours until the patient has recovered. Ice cubes held to the gluteal muscle before and after injection will reduce or eliminate pain and induration. When treatment continues for several days, the person can be placed on an ice cap between injections. When employing vitamin C intravenously, it is best to use sodium ascorbate and the solution free of all additives except sodium bisulfite. The dose of vitamin C using a syringe should range between 350 mg and 400 mg/kg body weight. In older patients or when very high doses are required, the vitamin can be added to 5 percent dextrose in water, in saline solution, or in a Ringer's solution. The concentration should be approximately 1 gram to 18cc fluid. Bottle injections will need 1 gram calcium gluconate one to two times each day to replace calcium ions removed by the high intravenous schedule. One quart of milk daily will suffice when using the vitamin intramuscularly. Or in the place of milk one can substitute calcium gluconate tablets. Supplemental vitamin C is always given by mouth. As a guide in determining the amount of frequency of injection we recommend our Silver Nitrate-Urine test. This is done by placing ten drops of 5 percent silver nitrate in a Wasserman tube and adding ten drops of urine. A color pattern will develop showing white, beige, smoke gray or one that looks like fine grain charcoal. Charcoal is the color needed and the test is performed at least every four hours. The test itself is read in one minute. . . . The killing power of vitamin C is not limited. When proper amounts are used it will destroy all virus organisms. . . . By 1950 we learned that we could kill the measles virus in 24 hours by giving intrasmuscular injections in a dose range of 350 mg/kg body weight every two hours. We also found that we could dry up chicken pox in the same time, but more dramatic results were obtained by giving 400 mg/kg body weight intravenously. In conclusion, the killing power of ascorbic acid on virus bodies has been demonstrated by me in hundreds of cases, many of which were treated in our hospital with nothing but vitamin C.[20]

When a person has been taking large dosages of vitamin C for a few days or weeks or longer, the amount of this nutrient in his blood is such that if he suddenly stops taking high dosages of it, blood levels of ascorbic acid will be rapidly converted into other substances, and the concentration of vitamin C in the blood will become abnormally low. This "rebound effect,"[21] as Dr. Linus Pauling calls it, in turn decreases one's resistance to further infectious flareup. It is accordingly wise for one who has been on a large dosage of vitamin C to decrease the intake gradually over a week or two, rather than suddenly. When decreasing vitamin C dosages, bowel tolerance levels should be maintained until you feel 100 percent well. Then continue to take your daily prophylactic dose of the nutrient.

In order for us really to appreciate the healing powers of vitamin C, we should look briefly at some of the firsthand clinical cases in which this nutrient was given in large dosages. Dr. Cathcart gives us some excellent examples of these clinical situations in which pneumonia, mononucleosis and hepatitis—illnesses so severe that traditional medical techniques such as the use of antibiotics can often take as long as a month or more to rehabilitate the patient—are effectively treated with vitamin C in less than a week. Of course, the patients must continue to take their individually determined bowel tolerance levels of vitamin C for some time or until they feel 100 percent better. But, basically, their severe symptoms are gone in three to five days after taking vitamin C in large dosages and they are able to continue their daily living patterns.

PNEUMONIA

Let me give you a typical case of a woman here, about 28, who developed viral pneumonia. As far as I could tell she did not respond to antibiotics and she never did "culture" any place. When she presented herself she was very ill, had a high temperature, the right upper lobe was infiltrated with the pneumonia process, and she had difficulty breathing. So we hooked her up to intravenous ascorbic acid, about 1 gram per 18 cc's and ran it in just as fast as we could. I gave her about 55 grams by vein and the remainder orally; about 215 grams went into her between 11 o'clock in the morning and 9 o'clock that night, at which time the pneumonia went into crisis. She drenched three sets of bed clothing that night. The next morning she was feeling much better. We did the same thing the next day. She returned to work less than a week after I saw her. We have daily X rays that demonstrate the rapid dissolution of the pneumonia process.

At that time I treated two other people in town who had the same thing, and got similar results. Three other patients in town went to other physicians and were hospitalized about two weeks and weren't much better when they came out. . . .

MONONUCLEOSIS

The first patient that I ran into with mononucleosis was a junior high school librarian who was about 22 and weighed about 100 pounds wringing wet. She came in with a severe case of mononucleosis. I told her about the bowel tolerance idea and explained to her how to do this self-titration. I saw her three or four days later; she was almost completely well. . . . The typical patient who gets mononucleosis is exactly the one who does the best on vitamin C: older teenagers or young adults are just fantastic vitamin C takers. They can understand the bowel tolerance idea, have iron stomachs, and couldn't care less about slight gas and diarrhea when they have this horrible disease. In fact the sicker the [patients are] the better [they do] because the relief of symptoms is so dramatic that they don't need any arguments to convince them to continue treatment. So what usually happens is that in three to five days the symptoms are 90 percent relieved. Then they must get the message loud and clear: if they stop the vitamin C too soon they get sick all over again.

HEPATITIS

The other disease that is very specific is infectious hepatitis. It's a cinch for vitamin C. The difference between the course of the disease with and without vitamin C is quite obvious if only because hepatitis is a disease that we can put numbers on. There are various enzyme systems that we can follow to show the course of the disease. Infectious hepatitis can be mild where the patient is just a little yellow and maybe a bit tender in the abdomen, but not very sick. But the patients I'm talking about— 20 of them, at least— were profoundly ill with hepatitis, and here again we were able to detoxify them in three to five days. The patient is feeling essentially well in three to four days. It generally takes about six days for the jaundice to clear. In two to three days the urine returns to normal color.

Hepatitis is a very serious problem, especially following blood transfusions. The whole system of gathering blood in this country is undergoing a revision because people who sell their blood have a high incidence of hepatitis. One of the most important clinical observations concerning prevention of hepatitis after transfusions was made by two Japanese physicians. Drs. Murata and Morishige discovered that an intake of more than 2 grams a day of vitamin C protects surgical patients who receive blood transfusions against serum hepatitis. There was about a 7 percent hepatitis level in their hospital. Then over 1100 patients

in the hospital were given 2 grams of vitamin C daily. The
physicians in charge expected at least 70 of the 1100 to develop
hepatitis—but not a single patient developed the viral disease
after having taken the vitamin C.[22]

As previously discussed, infections are a very important
link in the chain of events which makes up the diabetic
biochemical disease process. Infections weaken the biochemical system enough to create more serious nutritional
deficiencies and thus more severe allergic sensitivity. The
infections the patient is harboring, therefore, should always be a part of the differential diagnosis of possible
causes of symptoms, both physical and mental. Vitamin C
is obviously only one Bio-Ecologic method by which
infectious invasion can be controlled. An optimum supply
of all the other nutrients is needed as well: amino acids,
minerals and other vitamins. Vitamin B6 and pantothenic
acid, for example, are very important in dealing with the
stress of infectious disease.

Before concluding this chapter on vitamin C, we should
direct our attention toward specific criticisms of the use
and the "abuse" of large dosages of the nutrient. One of
these criticisms centers on the relationship existing between the formation of kidney stones and the taking of large
amounts of ascorbic acid. First of all, we should understand that kidney stones are of varying types. The
tendency to form kidney stones of the ordinary type,
phosphate stones, is actually lessened by keeping the urine
acid. Vitamin C, of course, can accomplish this very easily
and effectively. However, the *Medical Letter* and *Consumer
Reports* have written that persons with a tendency to form
kidney stones of the urate and cystine types should at all
times keep their urine alkaline.

These two specific reports further point out that vitamin
C might increase the chances of causing these stones to
form because of its tendency to make the urine more acid.
In such rare cases, ascorbic acid should not be eliminated
entirely; rather, it should merely be changed in its form.
That is, ascorbic acid is in fact alkaline if the sodium

ascorbate form of the nutrient is used. This alkaline form of
vitamin C is just as effective in treatment as the acid form
is; the only difference is that it will make the urine alkaline,
and materially reduce the chances of developing kidney
stones for patients with such a tendency.

Concern has also developed in the orthodox medical
community over the possibility of increasing the amount of
oxalic acid in the urine as a result of taking large amounts
of vitamin C. All of us normally excrete a small amount of a
substance called oxalate everyday. However, when large
quantities of oxalate are excreted, calcium oxalate kidney
stones can be formed. And it is true that a few people who
take large amounts of vitamin C start to produce abnormally
high levels of oxalate, which is then excreted by the
kidneys. The normal level of oxalate production is around
40 mg or less per twenty-four hours. This can rise very
quickly with an increased intake of vitamin C to 300 or 400
mg, which is definitely too high. Is this then sufficient
reason for stopping our intake of larger than RDA doses of
vitamin C? The answer to this question is an emphatic *no*.
The researchers who did the studies on levels of oxalate and
vitamin C intake were not aware of the fact that vitamin
B6 will actually *prevent* vitamin C induced oxalate
formation.

There was a patient who, when he began taking 8
grams of vitamin C daily, discovered that his oxalate level
skyrocketed from around 40 mg to 383 mg. When he
learned of this, he became very depressed because he
thought he would have to stop taking the nutrient. He
knew from past experiences that vitamin C at bowel tolerance levels had offered him many advantages. His conflict
was immediately ended upon a physician's recommendation
to take 50 mg of vitamin B6 twice daily along with his 8
grams of vitamin C. When he did this, his urinary oxalate
test, after only two weeks of such treatment, dropped to a
little less than 57 mg. Vitamin B6 had saved the day! Our
patient was also very happy to discover that he could
actually take up to 1500 mg of vitamin C by itself without

suffering an increase in his urinary oxalate excretion levels.

One other criticism that has been used as a reason for not taking large doses of vitamin C is that such an intake destroys the levels of vitamin B12 in the body. This reasoning was presented by Victor Herbert, M.D., and was based on his laboratory experiment done in 1974. But as a team of researchers have clearly demonstrated in 1979, Dr. Herbert's methodology used in arriving at his false conclusions was inaccurately and unscientifically conceived. For as this more recent—and more accurate—evidence states in the *Journal of the American Medical Association:*

> *Marcus, et al., showed that when an adequate amount of cyanide was present in the extraction step, previous incubation of a cottage cheese meal at 37 degrees C. for 30 minutes in the presence of 20 times the ascorbic acid (vitamin C) concentration used by Herbert and Jacob did not destroy the vitamin B12 in the meal. . . . Appropriate assay methods for vitamin B12 demonstrate that it is not destroyed by ascorbic acid in a mimicked gastric environment. . . . Herbert's previous report suggested degradation of vitamin B12 under these conditions, but this was apparently caused by incomplete protection of the extracted vitamin B12 in the assay procedure. If incubation at 37 degrees C. for 30 minutes is a laboratory mimic of the gastric environment, one must conclude that high doses of ascorbic acid do not affect the stability of vitamin B12 in vivo.[23]*

Based on these more accurate findings, it is appropriate to conclude that researchers like Herbert should be more careful and thoughtful in their experimental methodologies. Accurate experimental conclusions based on valid scientific laboratory testing is a necessity in order to protect the public's conceptions concerning nutrition and the field of Bio-Ecologic Medicine.

In conclusion, there are two fundamental nutritional rules that should be the foundation upon which a research study concerning nutrients and their actions in the body is built. First we must always keep in mind biochemical individuality when making any scientific studies. What is true for one person biochemically speaking might not at all be true for another, even if they are of the same age, sex and general health pattern. Each person is an individual and reacts individually to every event. In the case of the patient previously mentioned, he could tolerate 1500 mg of vitamin C daily without suffering an increase in his urinary oxalate excretion. You, however, might be able to tolerate ten times that amount. It all depends on biochemical individuality. This principle was already recognized more than twenty years ago in the *Heinz Handbook of Nutrition:*

> *Individual organisms differ in their genetic makeup and differ also in morphologic and physiologic aspects, including their endocrine activity, metabolic efficiency, and nutritional requirements. . . . It is often taken for granted that the human population is made up of individuals who exhibit average physiologic requirements and that a minor proportion of this population is composed of those whose requirements may be considered to deviate excessively. Actually there is little justification in nutritional thinking for the concept that a representative prototype of Homo sapiens is one who has average requirements with respect to all essential nutrients and thus exhibits no unusually high or low needs. In the light of contemporary genetic and physiologic knowledge and the statistical interpretations thereof, the typical individual is more likely to be one who has average needs with respect to many essential nutrients but who also exhibits some nutritional requirements for a few essential nutrients which are far from average.*[24]

This statement, unfortunately, has not been generally accepted by the medical establishment. Bio-Ecologic physicians, however, are making a serious attempt not only to discover more about the general ranges of human needs, but also to determine specifically for individuals what needs they may have which are far from average.

The second rule of nutrition that was reaffirmed by our study is known as the teamwork principle. Roger Williams was the first scientist to emphasize this rule. Simply stated, it means that nutrients never act by themselves in the body, but always function together as a team. Dr. Williams describes his principle in more detail:

The fourth basic fact in nutrition which has been sadly neglected by medical science is that of the essential "teamwork" among nutrients. Because this principle has been neglected, a wholly unscientific concept has been widely accepted with respect to what a nutrient may be expected to do.

The basic error, tacitly accepted, may be expressed as follows. Nutrients—amino acids, minerals, and particularly vitamins—are potential "medicines," and should be tested accordingly, using statistical methods and suitable placebo controls to determine their efficacy in combating diseases. If they prove to be "specifics" for particular diseases, well and good; if not, they must be regarded as medically worthless. . . . Following this erroneous reasoning, it is concluded that since specific individual nutrients are ineffective when tested in this way against specific common ailments, these nutrients are worthless for combating disease. It is easy to conclude also that there should be no substantial concern regarding the intake of these nutrients on the part of the patients.

The joker in the argument is that while no nutrient by itself is an effective remedy for any common disease, the nutrients acting as a team are probably effective in the prevention of a host of diseases. . . .

It must be emphasized that adequate nutrition must involve the complete chain of nutrients. If a diet is missing one link in the nutritional chain, it may be as worthless for supporting life as if it were missing 10 links. One nutrient, i.e., mineral, amino acid, or vitamin, added as a supplement to a food can bring no favorable effect unless the food contains some of all the other nutrients or unless they are available from the reserves of the person being nourished.[25]

Drugs are chemical substances which, even if given singularly, radically alter man's metabolic machinery and many times interfere with normal vitamin, mineral, amino acid and enzyme activities in the body. Nutrients, on the other hand, working as a team, act constructively as building blocks for life in general; without them human life could not exist. Life can exist without drugs! Nutrients, therefore, are not drugs and really should not be researched one at a time. In the case of our patient who formed calcium oxalate kidney stones, it would have been wrong to advise him, based on the clinical research concerning the single study of vitamin C and oxalate levels in the urine, never to take an increased amount of ascórbic acid. The supplement of vitamin B6 immediately stopped this rare occurrence of the formation of calcium oxalate kidney stones. In the experiment with vitamin B12 and vitamin C as described by Herbert in 1974, there was an "incomplete protection of the extracted vitamin B12 in the assay procedure," and this unscientific oversight led to false conclusions concerning the interactions of these two nutrients. Therefore, research must in the future take into account all the interactions of the different nutrients before any scientific conclusions are made.

We also must remember that no one nutrient cures anything by itself—even vitamin C. While vitamin C does have many positive effects in the battle against infectious and degenerative diseases, it alone, without all the other nutrients being supplied on an individually determined basis, is practically worthless. So remember, all nutrients are always team players. Every kind of organism derives its sustenance from food supplies containing teams of nutrients. The teamwork principle has, therefore, a very long history; it has been in action consistently and universally ever since life began on earth, and still governs our biochemical being.

REFERENCES

1. King, C. G. 1936. The relationship of vitamin C to Glucose tolerance in the guinea pig. *Journal of Biological Chemistry* 116:489–492.

2. Banerjee, S. 1943. Vitamin C and carbohydrate metabolism. *Nature* 152:152; Banerjee, S. 1943. Vitamin C and carbohydrate metabolism. *Annals of Biochemistry and Experimental Medicine* 3:157–164; Banerjee, S. 1964. Effect of scurvy on active transport of glucose by small intestine in vitro. *Proceedings Society Experimental Biology and Medicine* 116:216–218.12½

3. Banerjee, S. 1947. Relation of scurvy to glucose tolerance test. *Journal of Biological Chemistry* 168:207–211.

4. Altenburger, E. 1936. Relationship of ascorbic acid on the storage and metabolism of glycogen in the liver. *Klinische Wochenschrift* 15:1129–1131.

5. *Medical World News*, April 20, 1973.

6. Rogoff, J. M. 1944. Vitamin C and insulin action. *Pennsylvania Medical Journal* 47:579–582.

7. Pfleger, R. 1937. Diabetes and vitamin C. *Weiner Archiv für innere Medizin* 31:219–229.

8. *Medical World News*, April 5, 1974, p. 61.

9. Stone, I. 1972. *The Healing Factor: Vitamin C Against Disease*. New York: Grosset and Dunlap, p. 103.

10. *Ibid.*

11. Williams, R. J. 1973. *Nutrition Against Disease*. New York: Bantam Books, p. 262.

12. Sokoloff, B. 1966. *Journal of the American Geriatric Society* 14:1239.

13. Smolenskii, V. S. 1959. *Nauch. Akad. Nauk. Inst. Biokkim* 4:158.

14. Krall, L. 1978. *Joslin Diabetes Manual*, 11th ed. Philadelphia: Lea and Febiger, p. 179.

15. Williams, R. J. and Kalita, D. K. 1977. *A Physician's Handbook on Orthomolecular Medicine*. New Canaan, CT.: Keats Publishing, p. 46.

16. *Ibid.*, p. 46.

17. *Executive Health*. 1975. 12:3.

18. Stone, I. *The Healing Factor.*

19. *The Linus Pauling Newsletter*. Fall 1978, 1:4.

20. Williams, R. J. and Kalita, D. K. *A Physician's Handbook on Orthomolecular Medicine*, p. 52.

21. Pauling, L. 1976. *Vitamin C and the Common Cold*. San Francisco: Freeman and Company, pp. 115–118.

22. *The Linus Pauling Newsletter* 1:4.

23. *Journal of the American Medical Association*. November 23, 1979, pp. 2319–2320.

24. Burton, B. T., ed. 1959. *The Heinz Handbook of Nutrition*. New York: McGraw Hill.

25. Williams, R. J. and Kalita, D. K. *A Physician's Handbook on Orthomolecular Medicine*, p. 7.

CHAPTER EIGHT

Vitamin E and diabetic cardiovascular disease

The significance of vitamin E as an essential nutrient functioning in relation to diabetes is not, as might be expected, in the control of high blood sugar levels in the body. The rotation diet coupled with the use of proteolytic enzymes and amino acids successfully accomplishes this. Rather, vitamin E centers its healing powers on the very serious cardiovascular end product of the diabetic disease process. As Evan Shute, M.D., medical director of the famed Shute Institute, wrote:

> We think that no diabetic is being treated unless he is getting vitamin E. Diabetes is really two diseases, one disease being hyperglycemia. The blood sugar goes up, and the patient is controlled by diet and/or insulin. . . . All that does, as Joslan said many years ago, is to save the man from dying of hyperglycemia to let him die later of vascular disease. Fifty years after Banting and insulin, diabetes is still third on the list of causes of death. Banting did not conquer diabetes at all. He just relieved people temporarily of their hyperglycemic symptoms to let them die of arteriosclerosis. . . . Diabetes is still an uncon-

*trolled monster. Parenthetically, we found that when giving
vitamin E, 25 percent of our clinical diabetics who were on
insulin had a decrease of insulin requirement of ten units or
more. These decreases can occur suddenly, within the first
seventy-two hours of the initiation of treatment. We caution all
diabetics on insulin who begin to take vitamin E to carry some
candy in their pockets for fear they will have a prompt reaction
(low blood sugar), in the first two or three days. The insulin they
have needed for twenty-five years may suddenly become much
less. We have seen people taking as much as seventy units go off
of it entirely with the introduction of vitamin E; this does not
occur often, but we have seen it. As such, vitamin E occasionally
lowers insulin requirements; but that's not the big thing. The
important thing is that vitamin E looks after the vascular end of
cardiovascular disease. It saves eyes before they start to blow
up, and it saves gangrene before it starts. I don't see why people
have to wait until they stumble and fall before they try to pick
themselves off the ground. Why do people have to go on to
gangrene and all that sort of thing, and then call us in great
distress?*[1]

The answer, of course, to this unsettling question is
the fact that we Americans have fallen into the trap of
believing in "crisis medicine." The philosophy of crisis
medicine waits until symptomatic distress is extremely
active; the physician practicing this type of care then
rushes in—usually with some sort of drug therapy—to
temporarily relieve the current symptomatic complaint
(toximolecular medicine) of the patient. In our case, a good
example of this would be a physician giving only insulin
to diabetics while ignoring all other aspects of treating the
patient. By doing this, he obviously fails to understand the
dietary nutritional causes of the disease process he is
treating, and therefore overlooks the all important preventive—
long term—aspects of possible treatment modalities.

One of these preventive modalities in the treatment of
diabetes is the therapeutic use of vitamin E. As Dr. Shute
put it, vitamin E "looks after the vascular end of cardiovascular disease." Needless to say, the cardiovascular problems
associated with diabetes are today probably the most
important part of the disease process to understand—and

thus to cure. Unfortunately, in the past, they have been the least understood due to the sad fact that toximolecular crisis oriented physicians have been looking in the wrong direction for a possible cure. Be this as it is, vitamin E can be used as an effective weapon in preventing the long term diabetic cardiovascular complications. The reasons for this claim are fourfold: 1. vitamin E is a powerful *antioxidant;* 2. vitamin E is also reported to have a significant *anticlotting* effect and thus acts as a natural antithrombin; 3. vitamin E actually prevents myocardial scarring; 4. vitamin E can act as a *vasodilator* by opening unused blood vessels and strengthening heart performance.

In order to see how vitamin E helps to control diabetic cardiovascular complications, let us first examine one of its major functions: namely vitamin E as an antioxidant. As an antioxidant it improves the ability of our tissues to utilize oxygen. Accordingly, a vitamin E saturated blood system does not need as much oxygen to run efficiently as does a vitamin E deficient blood system. The implications of this in relation to allergy induced hyperglycemic reactions are noteworthy: As we have seen, maladaptive reactions usually reduce existing oxygen supplies in the body; by producing kinin as well as histamine (if immunologic) end products, these reactions use up necessary oxygen blood supplies. To see the importance of this in relation to diabetic cardiovascular complications, it is necessary to first understand that cholesterol often accumulates in various arteries at sites having low oxygen concentrations. If arteries to the heart are blocked by such cholesterol accumulations, the heart tissue dies due to oxygen starvation (i.e., infarct). But vitamin E helps to prevent both of these situations from occurring: by making red blood cells more efficient in utilizing life-giving oxygen, it simultaneously helps to minimize cholesterol buildup in potentially oxygen deficient tissues as well as increases the oxygen utilization efficiency of the heart. Consequently, by reducing the need for oxygen and increasing the efficiency of oxygen utilization, vitamin E dramatically increases the diabetic's chance for a healthy life free of cardiovascular complications.

Clinical findings support the assertion that vitamin E is a powerful antioxidant. As Roger J. Williams, Ph.D., writes:

Alpha tocopherol (vitamin E) has been credited with permitting the heart muscle to use oxygen more effectively. For this reason, it is of special merit for heart patients (De Nicola P. Inter. Cong. Vit. E, 1955). Death from a heart attack due to a clot or occlusion is the result of a shutting off of the oxygen supply. In his address to the International Congress on vitamin E in 1955, Evan Shute reported that much less of the heart tissue is destroyed during an attack if alpha tocopherol has been adequately supplied, and the patient is much more likely to survive the attack. . . . Shute's interpretation is that vitamin E functions best to conserve oxygen. Houshin and Mattill report that the oxygen need of the cardiac muscle is reduced by as much as 43 percent when vitamin E is administered (J. Biol. Chem., 146:309, 313, 1942). This may allow the amount of oxygen of the narrow stream of blood of the coronary artery reaching the heart to be adequate, in many patients, in preventing anoxia, thus preventing angina.[2]

As an effective antioxidant, vitamin E prevents unsaturated fatty acids and fatlike substances from being destroyed or made rancid by oxygen. Unless there are adequate levels of vitamin E present, oxygen will actually turn such polyunsaturated fats like corn oil, safflower oil and other vegetable oils in the body cells rancid by a process called peroxidation. In the raw state, these particular types of polyunsaturated fats contain enough vitamin E to prevent peroxidation from occurring, but the oils on our grocery shelves today are all too often deficient in vitamin E, due to the boiling, deodorizing, processing, refining and bleaching of them by the food processors. Peroxidation, biochemically speaking, is an inflammatory process: when it occurs, substances called free radicals are simultaneously produced. Free radicals are very toxic substances which move around in the cells of our bodies with terrific force and without any distinguishable pattern. They usually end up striking a molecule within the cell, which may cause serious damage. Inflammatory damage such as this within the blood vessel walls occurs when these highly reactive chemical fragments called free radicals react with the walls. However, vitamin E deactivates free radicals by sacrificing itself to them—thus destroying the free radicals. If vitamin E is not present to deactivate the free radicals produced by peroxidation of polyunsaturated oils, the free radical reactions produce severe irritations on active sites within the cell wall, and thus the arteriosclerotic disease process begins.

The implications of this line of reasoning are indeed very serious. The popular fad of today is to consume more polyunsaturated fatty acids (corn oils, margarines) than saturated fats. But the trouble with this proposition is that it overlooks the important ratio needed between the consumption of too much polyunsaturated fatty acids and too little vitamin E. "This situation," writes Dr. Roger J. Williams, "if true, is indeed ironical: Current popular proposals to prevent arteriosclerosis in coronary heart disease virtually ignore the nutritional balance of cellular environments; consequently, their advocacy of more polyunsaturated fatty acids in the diet may actually be accelerating cardiovascular mortality in our population, while creating a nutritional vitamin E deficiency."[3]
Dr. Williams arrives at this conclusion through the following steps of reasoning and by examining the following clinical studies:

Polyunsaturated fatty acids, particularly linoleic acid, are, of course, easily oxidized. From numerous studies of poultry, rats, rabbits, cattle, and man, investigators have found that increased ingestion of polyunsaturated fats requires greater amounts of antioxidants in the diet, particularly vitamin E. (See Horwitt, M.K. Am. J. Clin. Nutr., 4:408, 1956; Ibid. 8:451, 1960; Hove, E.L., and Harris, P.L. J. Nutr., 33:95, 1947; Dam, H. Proc. Soc. Exp. Biol. Med., 52:285, 1953; Century, B., and Horwitt, M.K. J. Nutr., 72:357, 1960; Filer, L.J., Jr., et al. In Trans. First Conf. Biol. Antioxidants, New York: Macy, 1946, pp. 67–77; Witting, L.A., and Horwitt, M.K. J. Nutr., 82:19, 1964; Horwitt, M.K., et al. J. Am. Dietet. Assoc., 38:231, 1961; Harris, P.L. and Embree, N.D. Am. J. Clin. Nutr., 13:385, 1963; Hassan, H., et al. Am. J. Clin. Nutr.,

19:147, 1966; Ritchie, J., et al. Proc. Soc. Pediat. Res., Apr. 1967, p. 107; Blaxter, K.L., et al. Brit. J. Nutr., 7:287, 1953.)

Increasing polyunsaturated fats in the diet appears to augment the amount of vitamin E needed daily (Horwitt, M.K., Borden's Rev. Nutr. Res., 22:1, 1961; Council on Foods and Nutrition. JAMA 181–411, 1962). Horwitt and his associates found that in man the higher the unsaturated fats in the diet, the lower was the tocopherol in the plasma (J. Am. Dietet. Assoc., 38:231, 1961). Tocopherol requirements, they determined, will vary from 5 milligrams to 30 milligrams or more per day, depending on the amount of polyunsaturated fatty acids in the diet.

Lipid peroxidation may be important with respect to cellular aging. A. L. Tappel has presented evidence that implicates polyunsaturated fatty acids as being the primary source of free peroxy radicals that damage the cellular membranes (endoplasmic reticulum and mitochondria) and accelerate aging (Nutr. Today, 2:2, 1967). Tappel points out that if the intake of polyunsaturated fatty acids exceeds the intake of nutrient anti-oxidants (such as vitamin E and selenium, a trace antioxidant) required for their stability in the body, the condition will be dangerously productive of lipid peroxidation (Geriatrics, 23:97, 1968; Fed. Proc., 24:73, 1965).

W. S. Hartroft and E. A. Porta describe the morbid condition of ceroid pigment deposition in animal and human tissues (Am. J. Med. Scie., 250:324, 1965). This pigment is classified as a lipochrome, similar to such pigments as found, for instance, in the muscle of experimental nutritional muscular dystrophy. Authorities in this area of research appear to agree that ceroid pigment results from "oxidation and peroxidation of polyunsaturated fats with the formation of long-chain polymers of an insoluble nature" (Hartroft, W. S., and Porta, E. A. "Present Knowledge of Ceroid Pigments." In Present Knowledge in Nutrition, New York: The Nutrition Foundation, 1967; Endicott, K.M. Arch. Path., 37:49, 1944; DeOlivera, J. D. Ann. N.Y. Acad. Sci., 52:125, 1949–1950; Dam, H., and Granadox, H. Science, 103:327, 1945).

Ceroid pigment formation has been reported in man to be a relatively early and constant condition in atherosclerotic aortas and coronary arteries "as well as in occlusive thrombi found obstructing the latter in cases of fatal myocardial infarction" (Hartroft and Porta, op. cit.). Hartroft and Porta note that vitamin

E and other antioxidants will decrease the formation of ceroid pigment. (See also Tappel, A. L. Arch. Biochem., 54:266, 1955.)

They also state, "It is apparent . . . that the nutritional status of the entire organism may play an important role in whether or not ceroid will be deposited in any part of the body. A high intake of polyunsaturated fat or a low intake of vitamin E (and particularly the simultaneous presence of both conditions), will favor its formation, particularly if abnormal deposits of lipids form in liver, muscle, or other organs."

SUMMARY: Briefly, we have reviewed data which indicate that, (1) a high polyunsaturated fatty acid intake may cause a critical shortage of vitamin E in the system unless additional tocopherols are included in the diet; (2) if additional antioxidants (vitamin E, selenium, vitamin C) are not included in a high unsaturated fat diet, it may be dangerously productive of lipid peroxidation and, hence, cellular aging; (3) if additional antioxidants are not provided (specifically alpha tocopherol), a high polyunsaturated fat diet may promote ceroid pigment formation which has been found in atherosclerotic aortas and coronary arteries in man. Moreover, these ceroid pigments (containing polyunsaturated fatty acids) found in occlusive thrombi or clots are more resistant to dissolution than those clots containing saturated fat.

If the above indictments are correct, it is suggested that individuals who ingest a large amount of polyunsaturated fats on the notion that it will protect them against atherosclerosis and coronary heart disease may actually be exposing themselves to the disease! It may well be that one of the main reasons why Evan Shute and his colleagues have had such success with mega-alpha tocopherol therapy in a considerable number of coronary cases is because of our excessive intake of polyunsaturated fats in the last three decades, creating a vitamin E deficiency in numerous members of our population.[4]

The second major preventive function of vitamin E in the battle against cardiovascular disease is its effective anticlotting powers. Many clinicians have discovered alpha tocopherol's natural anticlotting effect in the blood (Mason, K.E. The Yale Journal for Biological Medicine., 14:605, 1942; Ames, S. R. Inter. Rev. Vit. Res., 22–41, 1951). Indeed, one researcher went so far as to state that in his view as a medical doctor, vitamin E's effectiveness as an anticlotting agent in the blood is greater in this regard than are the anticoagulant drugs, and is so without their dangerous side effects (Suffel, P. *Canad. Med. Assoc. J.*, 74:715, 1956). The reason for this is that vitamin E is a natural antithrombin, which circulates in the blood of all people, and prevents undue clotting; it does not interfere with the normal process of blood clotting as in the case of a wound. In fact, it is reported to enhance and actually shorten the time of healing burns and wounds (Zierlar, M. *N. Y. Acad. Sci.*, 52, 180, 1949).

Any trained physician knows that thrombin is an enzyme present in the blood serum that reacts with a complex protein of the globulin group known as fibrogen. This chemical reaction then forms fibrin, an insoluble protein that promotes the clotting of blood. Vitamin E is a natural antithrombin agent that in effect prevents the clotting of arteries but does not cause—as do some drugs—hemorrhaging. "Vitamin E," writes Alton Ochsner, M.D., of the Ochsner Clinic in New Orleans, "is an efficient antithrombic agent, and is probably one of the principal antithrombins in the blood. By supplying antithrombin in the form of vitamin E, the deficiency in antithrombin is corrected and a clot is prevented. The great advantage of using vitamin E is that although the thrombosing tendency is overcome, a hemorrhagic (bleeding) tendency is not produced, such as occurs when anticoagulants, for instance, heparin or dicumarol, are used."[5]

Obviously any natural anticlotting (antithrombic) effect in relation to arteriosclerosis is very important, since a clot in the coronary arteries can produce an infarct which will usually result in severe heart damage or even death; likewise, a clot in the cerebral arteries leading to the brain produces a stroke. Any natural preventive nutrient or combination of nutrients that can eliminate such clotting effects is a very valuable medical tool that deserves our utmost attention. Almost without exception, this is the reason why medical doctors should be researching nutrient therapy in relation to diabetic arteriosclerosis. For as we have clearly seen, vitamin B6 helps eliminate arterial lesion formation. Vitamin C strengthens the arterial walls by aiding in the formation of the structural cement known as collagen. This action prevents rupture and bleeding within the arterial walls. And now we learn that vitamin E significantly reduces the chances of any blood clot formation in the arteries and also increases the more effective use of oxygen. As a natural antithrombin, it is a very desirable and effective treatment modality, since death from heart attack is usually a result of a blood clot that shuts off an adequate blood supply carrying life giving oxygen. All this is why, if one can 1. eliminate the developing arterial lesions (B6); 2. strengthen the arterial wall and avoid rupture and bleeding (vitamin C); and finally 3. increase the body's effective use of available oxygen as well as prevent arterial clotting, heart attacks due to diabetic arteriosclerosis will be avoided to a much greater degree than if these essential nutrient functions are not present and working in the body.

The third major preventive function of vitamin E in the battle against cardiovascular disease is its ability to reduce any harmful overproduction of scar tissue. When an individual survives a myocardial infarct, usually the oxygen-starved tissue dies. In turn, the dead tissue then stimulates the creation of scar tissue. Scarring is a preventive measure of the body; its fundamental purpose is to prevent an infarcted area from rupturing. Large scars near the heart or in the heart obviously weaken that central organ's function. Vitamin E helps recovery from an infarct by minimizing tissue death from oxygen starvation and by reducing excessive scarring. Research and experimental studies with vitamin E substantiate these ideas. As Roger Williams states:

> Both Zierler of Johns Hopkins and Kay of Tulane have reported that alpha tocopherol, under normal conditions, is a natural antithrombin which circulates in the blood of all people, and prevents undue clotting; but it does not interfere with the normal process of blood clotting in the case of a wound (Zierler, M., et al. Ann. N.Y. Acad. Sci., 52:180, 1949; Kay, J.H., Surgery, 28:124, 1950). In fact, it is said to enhance and shorten the time of healing in burns and wounds.
>
> Madsen first showed that myocardial scarring was promoted

in vitamin E deficient rats (J. Nutr., 11:471, 1936). Later Mason and Emmels corroborated this early finding while reporting gross cardiac enlargement in autopsied rats (Anat. Rec., 92:33, 1945). After about the tenth to twelfth month of vitamin E deficiency in the rat, these investigators observed the appearance of pigment globules in "cardiac muscle fibers, usually as linear groups located irregularly in the sarcoplasm but sometimes as small clusters at each role of the nucleus resembling 'brown atropy' in man." After a year on an E deficient diet, definite histological injury to the cardiac muscle was apparent, with the peripheral portion of the ventricles showing the "most marked lesions." Autopsies of rats on a long term E deficient diet showed gross evidence of cardiac enlargement or dilatation.

A.J. Gatz and O.B. Houchin reported similar findings in the hearts of E deficient rabbits (Anat. Rec., 97:337, 1946); W. Bragdon confirmed this in similar observations (Proc. Second Vitamin E. Confer., Columbia University, N. Y., Jan. 23, 1948).

As early as 1944, in a study of cardiac insufficiency in E deficient rats, Houchin and Smith concluded, from the evidence of severe myocardial damage, that the sudden death of the E deficient animals "in an advanced stage of muscular dystrophy is due directly to myocardial failure" (Am. J. Physiol., 141:242, 1944). Other studies corroborated these earlier findings (Martin, E.V., and Faust, F.B. "The heart in avitaminosis E." Exper. Med. & Surg., 5:455, 1947; Butturine, U. "The heart in avitaminosis E." Gior. di Clin. Med., 27:400, 1946).

During this same decade, other researchers reported heart lesions in E deficient monkeys, while in the macaque species, vascular damage was more predominant (Mason, K. E., and Telford, I. R. "Some manifestations of vitamin E deficiency in the monkey." Arch. Path., 63:363, 1947). Russell Holman's experiments with dogs revealed an association between E deficiency and arterial lesion (Proc. Soc. Exp. Biol. Med., 66:307, 1947). In twenty-two of the twenty-five dogs fed high fat diets (3.0 cubic centimeters/kilograms of cod liver oil daily), Holman found that vitamin E was "equally effective in preventing or retarding the arterial lesions when its administration by mouth was started 0, 1, and 2 days after renal insufficiency was induced."

Cattle fed E deficient rations were observed to have decreased functional activity of the heart in the terminal stages of E deficiency with atrophy and scarring of the cardiac muscle fibers (Gullickson, T., and Calverley, C. Science, 104:312, 1946). All of these cattle died prematurely, suddenly, apparently of myocardial infarction.[6]

The fourth major preventive cardiovascular function of vitamin E is its ability to open unused blood vessels, thus acting as a natural vasodilator. This assertion is based on Dr. Evan Shute's contention[7] that large dosages of vitamin E (alpha tocopherol) given victims of myocardial infarction actually opens unused blood vessels and thus aids in further protecting heart attack victims. A study done by South American investigators experimentally supports Dr. Shute's thinking: these investigators[8] first induced heart attacks in dogs by ligating a branch of the coronary artery. Then half of the dogs were given 10 mg of vitamin E (a small dose) while the other half were given no additional nutrient support. Upon autopsy, the vitamin E experimental dogs had a greater dilation of the vessels in the area of the infarction. In addition, there was microscopic evidence to suggest that the internal structures of the infarcted area in the dogs had an abundance of many new capillaries, increased vascularization in the coronary areas, due partly to the dilation of old vessels and partly to the formation of new ones. The vitamin E deficient animals manifested none of these encouraging results.

Based upon clinical as well as experimental evidence, it is now easy to see why so many physicians believe that vitamin E is a very important nutrient in relation to maintaining cardiovascular integrity, especially in the diabetic. It is a powerful antioxidant; it is a natural antithrombin; it prevents excessive scarring; and at the same time it acts as a vasodilator. All these life-giving functions are extremely important to the diabetic with arteriosclerosis. In this chapter we have spent considerable time on this one particular nutrient. But again, it is important to realize that all nutrients work best together as a team. Vitamin E by itself is no miraculous cure-all of heart attack victims or diabetics with arteriosclerosis. It is, however, one of the very essential ingredients needed for cardiovascular well-being. There are, of course, other nutrients that are equally important. One such nutrient is vitamin B1.

The integrity of the heart, both in its function and its structure, is dependent on nutrition. Obviously, the heart differs in no way from other tissues and/or organs in its need for proper nutritional support. Therefore, single or multiple deficiencies of the various essential nutrients, whether vitamins, amino acids or minerals, may be expected to have profound consequences on the heart. Although many of the earlier experiments dealing with the effects of vitamin B1 (thiamine) deficiency on the heart are open to criticism because other nutrients were lacking, it seems clear now that the integrity of the heart as well as all the arteries is dependent on the presence of this essential nutrient. Important experimental studies on the relation of the vitamin B1 and heart disease clearly reveal that vitamin B1 deficiency results in severe damage to the heart and arteries. Indeed, even death has been reported in thiamine deficient swine. On autopsy, microscopic lesions of the heart were described in these thiamine deficient animals.[9]

Folic acid is another nutrient which appears to be deficient in the cellular environment of arteriosclerosis. Seventeen elderly patients with arteriosclerosis were given 5 to 7.5 mg of folic acid daily.[10] Fifteen of the seventeen patients responded favorably to the treatment: There was increased capillary blood flow and improved vision. The improved vision was believed to be a result of a better supply to the retina, thus reversing to some degree the arteriosclerotic condition.

Other important observations have been reported when rats were placed on vitamin A deficient diets.[11] In 75 percent of the newborn rats conceived by the vitamin A deficient mother rats, some degree of heart malfunction was observed. The primary deficiency observed was a failure of the interventricular spectrum to close. The second defect was a general failure of normal heart development: aortic arch anomalies were frequently present.

We could continue our discussion by examining each and every vitamin and how a subsequent deficiency affects actual heart performance. But that is not the function of this chapter. Rather we concentrated on one specific nutrient, namely vitamin E, so as to give a detailed presentation of precisely how one nutrient is involved in cardiovascular integrity. Obviously, all the various vitamins play a role to some degree in that function. For a more detailed account of the many nutritional deficiencies possible, and the resulting malfunctions of the cardiovascular system, see Dr. Roger Williams's *Nutrition Against Disease*, pp. 671–91.

REFERENCES

1. Shute, E. S. Winter 1973. Vitamin E. *Journal of Applied Nutrition* 25(1):39–40.

2. Williams, R. J. 1973. *Nutrition Against Disease*. New York: Bantam Books, pp. 243–244.

3. ____. *Nutrition Against Disease*, p. 259.

4. ____. *Ibid*. pp. 257–258.

5. Ochsner, Alton. 1949. Vitamin E: an efficient antithrombin agent. *Surgery*.

6. Williams, R. J. *Nutrition Against Disease*, pp. 242–243.

7. Shute, E. S. 1942. *Obstetrics and Gynecology in the British Empire* 49:482.

8. Puente-Dominguez. 1956. *Summary* 8.

9. Wintrobe, M. M. et al. 1943. Electrocardiographic changes associated with thiamine deficiency in pigs. *Bulletin*, Johns Hopkins Hospital 73:169; Asburn, L. L. and Lowry, J. V. 1944. Development of cardiac lesions in thiamine-deficient rats. *Archives of Pathology* 32:27; Swank, R. L. et al. 1941. The production and study of cardiac failure in thiamine-deficient dogs. *American Heart Journal* 22:154; Toman, J. E. P. et al. 1945. Origin of cardiac disorders in thiamine-deficient cats. *Proceedings of the Society for Experimental Biology and Medicine* 58:65; Waisman, H. A. and McCall, K. B. 1944. A study of thiamine deficiency in the monkey (macaca mulatta). *Archives of Biochemistry* 4:265.

10. Kopjas, T. 1966. Effect of folic acid on collateral circulation in diffuse chronic arteriosclerosis. *Journal of the American Geriatric Society* 14:1187.

11. Wilson and Warkary. 1949. Aortic-arch and cardiac anomalies in the offspring of vitamin A deficient rats. *American Journal of Anatomy* 85:113.

CHAPTER NINE

Chromium and Diabetes

So far we have centered our attention on specific vitamins, amino acids and/or proteolytic enzymes and their relationships to diabetes and cardiovascular disease. Another very special nutrient which is intimately connected with diabetes is called chromium. As far back as 1957, researchers named Swartz and Mertz[1] recognized that chromium is a very important factor in maintaining proper glucose metabolism. At that time, they were studying dietary deficiency patterns in rats; one such deficiency pattern was an intolerance to glucose (i.e., diabetes). After running many tests, they discovered that the substance causing the observed intolerance to glucose was a chromium compound. This substance (i.e., 20–50 u of chromium per 100 grams of body weight) was given to deficient rats in later studies, done around 1959, by these two researchers; they found that the rats' tolerance to injected glucose was immediately restored upon being given this substance.[2] "Their pioneering discovery," writes Henry Schroeder, M.D., "in retrospect was to have one of the most important and far-reaching effects on the nutritional aspects of human disease in the mid-twentieth century. Later, Mertz showed conclusively that chromium was necessary for the utilization of insulin in glucose metabolism."[3]

Chromium is a micronutrient (i.e., trace element) which means deficiencies and/or excesses are measured in extremely small amounts. Be this as it may, it remains an extremely important nutrient, since even the slightest deficiency of this important nutrient upsets the body's proper tolerance to glucose. In 1974, when chromium was examined in more detail, it was reported by Mertz[4] that pure chromium (Cr) as it appears in food, water or nature is not an accurate measure of dietary chromium, as this inorganic chromium is poorly absorbed in the human body—as little as 3 percent. Furthermore, it appears that inorganic chromium does not cross the placenta barrier although the infant human has a higher level of chromium in his system than at any other time in life. The only type of chromium presently thought to be biologically active in the human body is a trivalent chromium. This form is commonly referred to as GTF; in this form, chromium is bound together with two niacin molecules (vitamin B3) and three separate free amino acids: glutamic acid, glycine and cysteine. This natural chromium complex is much better absorbed and utilized than are the single chromium salts.[5]

There is some evidence that GTF is stored in the liver and is mobilized in response to glucose loading or to the administration of insulin. "An interesting observation was reported by Glinsmann," writes Taher Fouad, Ph.D., "where a correlation was established between insulin concentration and chromium levels in the blood. An increase in serum, whether by injecting the hormone or by oral or parenteral administration by glucose, always leads to an accurate increase of serum chromium within thirty to one hundred and twenty minutes in normal people."[6] The interesting point here is the fact that an increased intake of either glucose and/or insulin simultaneously calls for a release of chromium GTF reserves in the body. But what significance does this fact have for people living in the United States? U.S. statistics show an extremely high intake of sugar (i.e., 120 grams average per person per day). Sugar not only contains almost no chromium, but usually leads to a loss of body chromium because of the depleting effect of glucose.[7] That is, when pure sugar (either sucrose or glucose) is fed in large amounts to a fasting person, three things happen to that individual. First, his blood sugar is elevated; second, insulin in the blood rises dramatically; and third, chromium in the blood increases, since it is mobilized from storage levels in the body tissues. The chromium in the blood, elevated in response to the sugar intake and the co-presence of insulin, then travels to the kidneys, where between 20 and 30 percent of the blood chromium is excreted in the urine. The result is a net loss of chromium in the body. The proof of all this comes from the documented evidence that diabetic individuals excrete chromium more rapidly in their urine than do people not having diabetes.[8] "In two separate studies," writes Dr. Fouad, "it was shown that in cases of severe chromium deficiencies, a syndrome similar to diabetes was observed in rats and mice. This syndrome was immediately reversed when five parts per million of chromium was added to the drinking water. It is, therefore, safe to assume that the primary biochemical lesion in chromium deficiency is manifested by the decreased sensitivity of the peripheral tissue to insulin. . . . Chromium exerts its action in the tissue not as an insulin-like agent, but as a true potentiator of the action of the hormone itself."[9]

Thus, all of this leads to a biochemically vicious circle in which the intake of either large amounts of sugar or the intake of insulin automatically causes a depletion of chromium; on the other hand, a deficiency of chromium causes an increased intolerance to glucose and therefore necessitates the injection of more and more insulin.

Carbohydrates other than white sugar may also be responsible for chromium deficiencies in the human body. All starches are digested into sugars in the intestines and then used for energy sources. In the United States, the

major source of carbohydrate calories other than white sugar
is refined white flour. Fortunately, wholewheat flour
contains 175 mg of chromium per 100 grams of wheat;
unfortunately, however, refined white flour—the "staple"
of the American diet— contains only 23 mg of chromium
per 100 grams of refined white flour. This same process by
which white sugar causes chromium depletion in the body
can occur with GTF deficient white bread. "Therefore, the
typical American diet," writes Henry Schroeder, M.D.,
"with about 60 percent of its calories taken from refined
sugar and refined flour, was apparently designed not only to
provide as little chromium as feasible, but to cause
depletion of body stores of chromium by not replacing
urinary loss. Again, the article of faith based on reason
stated previously, that whole foods contain the micronutrients (chromium and others) necessary for their proper
metabolism, has been shown to hold true, and the refining
of these foods based on custom, habit, preference, and
industrial practices, has been shown to provide foods
lacking in a significant amount of micronutrients necessary
for their metabolism."[10] It seems, therefore, that we Americans are bent on "refining" ourselves into a chromium
deficiency, the ultimate result of which is a significant
glucose intolerance in the human body. This rather unhappy
distinction of the United States is not shared by other countries
that do not refine their foods. In a series of tests on men
between the ages of twenty and fifty-nine, the amount of
chromium found in the heart artery was 1.9 parts per million
(ppm) in American men, 5.5 ppm in African men, 11 ppm in
men from the Near East, and 15 ppm in men in the Far East.
This evidence is one source of speculation which proves
that there is indeed a definite link between the over-
consumption of refined foods and a chromium deficiency.

Chromium and arteriosclerosis

At present there are not very many experimental studies
connecting arteriosclerosis to a chromium deficiency. One

interesting study done by Dr. Schroeder in 1960 strongly suggests that there may be some biochemical correlation between the development of arteriosclerotic plaques and chromium deficiency. In that year, Dr. Schroeder performed a comprehensive study on the effects of certain trace elements given to rats and mice from weaning until death. The elements lead, cadmium and chromium were the first three experimental substances used. Admittedly, Dr. Schroeder was not aware at that time how important chromium was in maintaining optimum human and animal health. It was decided that the control animals were to receive no chromium supplement and their diet was to contain as little as possible of it. As it turned out, the rats receiving dietary and supplemental chromium "grew faster, survived longer, and at death, surprisingly enough, had no arteriosclerotic plaque in their aortas."[11] The other animals receiving little or no dietary supplemental chromium had arteriosclerotic plaques in 20 percent of their aortas. These and other animals, about seven hundred of them in all, also had elevated blood cholesterol and sugar levels. As Dr. Schroeder summarizes:

> Taking all of these findings together, we could believe that we had reproduced in rats the human disorder in fat and sugar metabolism which leads to arteriosclerosis. The degree of severity of the disorder, however, was mild to moderate; the rat is one of the most typical animals to make arteriosclerotic, requiring extreme measures; we had done it without extreme measures, using ordinary foods, merely by introducing chromium deficiency, and prevented it with chromium. Other studies further corroborate this idea. Rats were given a diet of half white sugar, a third torula yeast (both low in chromium) and the rest lard. When chromium was given, cholesterol was slow and mild diabetes absent; without it, cholesterol and blood sugar were elevated.[12]

The significance of these animal studies becomes more apparent when one examines the statistical percentages of chromium deficiencies in American adults as compared with people in other less industrialized countries. Usually, babies and children up to ten years of age have relatively high levels of chromium present in their bodies, and this is true whether they are American or from other countries. But by the time American adults get to be over fifty years old, 23 percent have severe chromium deficiencies, whereas only 1.5 percent of adults in foreign countries manifest this essential element deficiency. Estimates, for example, based on organ weights indicate that Africans have twice, Near Easterners 4.4 times and Orientals 5 times as much chromium in their bodies as do Americans. Granted that we have no direct clinical evidence of chromium deficiency causing arteriosclerosis; but the fact remains that people who die of coronary artery disease (i.e., arteriosclerosis) have no detectable amount of chromium present in their aortas, while those who die accidentally, manifesting no coronary artery disease, do have chromium present in their aorta.

With this knowledge at hand, we must look to the day when this essential micronutrient is not, by a process of refining, removed from the major sources of our food supplies. Modern industrialized man has within his grasp the knowledge of preventive medicine; he also has within himself the seeds of self-destruction, when in the face of knowledge he flouts the wisdom of nature's commands for health and life.

REFERENCES

1. Swartz, K. and Mertz, W. 1957. *Archives of Biochemistry and Biophysics* 72:515.

2. ____. 1959. *Archives of Biochemistry and Biophysics* 82:292.

3. Schroeder, H. A. 1973. *The Trace Elements and Man.* Old Greenwich, Conn: Devin-Adair, p. 71.

4. Mertz, W.; Toepfer, W.; Rogimski, E. E.; and Polansky, M. M. 1974. Present knowledge of the role of chromium. 33:2275–2280.

5. ____. 1971. Newer trace elements in nutrition. *Federation Proceedings.* eds. Mertz and Cornatzer. New York: Dekker, p. 127.

6. Fouad, M. T. 1979. Chromium and diabetes. *Journal of Applied Nutrition* 31 (1 & 2):18.

7. Glinsman, W. H. 1966. *Science* 152:1243.

8. Doisy, R. S. 1971. Newer trace elements in nutrition, p. 155.

9. Fouad, M. T. Chromium and diabetes, p. 18.

10. Schroeder, H. A. *The Trace Elements and Man*, p. 78.

11. *Ibid.*, p. 72.

12. *Ibid.*

CHAPTER TEN

Cardiovascular disease and minerals

A researcher named Kobayashi[1] first suggested in 1957 that there is a relationship between the quality of water we drink and the number of deaths due to cardiovascular disease. These first insights correlating the quality of water and cardiovascular disease have been reviewed by many other researchers, and since then have been expanded in their scope and understanding. Schroeder, for example, reviewing data from the United States census of 1950, suggested that average statewide, age-adjusted annual death rates varied from a maximum of 983 per 100,000 people in South Carolina—a "soft-water" state—to a minimum of only 712 in Nebraska—a "hard-water" state.[2] In his analysis, deaths were divided into two fundamental groups: 1. cardiovascular, and 2. all others. In considering only the deaths related to the first category, Schroeder discovered that the percentage difference between states was much larger than the total death category; in fact, when he compared cardiovascular death rates in South Carolina (soft water) to New

Mexico (hard water), he was amazed to find that South Carolina had a 76 percent greater cardiovascular death rate than New Mexico! The figures were 511 in the soft water state as compared to 290 in the hard water state.

Other more recent studies confirm Schroeder's original work. Masironi compared death rates for people living near the basins of two hard water and two soft water rivers in the United States. Over 7 million people living in over 140 counties along the Ohio and Columbia (soft water) Rivers, and along the Missouri and Colorado (hard water) Rivers were compared and analyzed.[3] As expected, death rates from cardiovascular diseases were much lower in the hard water regions (i.e., near the Missouri and Colorado Rivers); in fact, they were 41 percent and 25 percent lower respectively as compared to the soft water Ohio and Columbia Rivers.

Even more convincing evidence comes from a study done on Monroe County, Florida in 1972.[4] The water supply of this particular county was suddenly changed from rain water, with a hardness of only 0.5 ppm to deep well water with a hardness of 200 ppm. Most people residing in Monroe County live on a chain of small islands dotting the map between the tip of Florida and Key West; accordingly, there are practically no other sources of water for these people. After the change to the harder water, the cardiovascular death rate dropped from the 600 to 700 range to the 200 to 300 range within four years!

What makes water hard, of course, is its content of such minerals as magnesium, zinc, iron, calcium, chromium, cobalt, copper, manganese, nickel, selenium, tin and so forth. Based on the evidence presented previously, we can logically conclude, therefore, that man's intake of specific minerals must affect in a very important way the health and integrity of his entire cardiovascular system; indeed, a balanced mineral intake is the foundation upon which every healthy cell—of which there are trillions in each of our cardiovascular systems—is constructed and sustained in life. If this is true, and every indication points to that very fact, then it behooves us to examine some of the specific minerals in order to see if there truly exists an empirical relationship between their intake into the human body and the prevention of cardiovascular disease.

One of the most important minerals needed for maintaining a healthy cardiovascular system—especially in the diabetic—is magnesium. The administration of magnesium in the successful treatment of cardiovascular diseases was tried as long ago as 1930 by Malkiel and Shapiro.[5] Parsons[6] in 1960 gave us more scientific data based on clinical biochemical findings which supports the previous researcher's views that magnesium therapy can be very beneficial in the treatment of cardiovascular disease. These researchers and others[7] believe that the proper administration of magnesium actually reduces total plasma lipids and serum cholesterol. They also believe that magnesium is an effective vasodilator. Brown suggests, and rightly so, that these results have been ignored by most medical clinicians.

R. J. Doisy presents an interesting and extremely competent study and discussion on the relationship existing between the death rate of diabetics with cardiovascular problems and the levels of magnesium and calcium in their drinking water. Writes Doisy:

> In a preliminary study that I carried out, water quality and the death rate due to diabetes was investigated in the state of Missouri. Since diabetes predisposes to vascular disease, a similar negative correlation between water hardness and the death rate due to diabetes might be anticipated. Using the published Vital Statistics for the State of Missouri for a ten year period (1960 through 1970), the crude death rate due to diabetes was determined for each county. The chemical composition of the water supplies for all cities, towns, and villages listed for a given county was weighted for the number of persons consuming water for a given water supply. The parameters considered were calcium and magnesium content and total hardness in ppm.
>
> Arbitrarily, the six counties with the highest death rate due to diabetes were compared to the six counties with the lowest death rate. . . . Five of six counties with the highest death rate were north of the Missouri River. Magnesium levels in the drinking water north of the river were lower than those south of the river, while calcium levels were similar in both regions.[8]

Obviously, such studies which base their evidence on correlation do not prove causation of the facts they are presenting. Doisy does present, however, convincing evidence as to the importance of magnesium and its relationship to maintaining cardiovascular health. He also suggests that proper calcium-magnesium ratios are extremely important to all diabetics. The reason for this assertion is based on the following thinking: There are a number of studies[9] done that offer evidence confirming that calcium, like magnesium, actually reduces circulating cholesterol levels in the blood. It has been known, however, that calcium and magnesium are antagonists. That is, if a diet is high in calcium and marginal in magnesium, a negative magnesium balance may ensue if the high calcium intake continues for any length of time. On the other hand, Hendrix[10] has shown that increasing the magnesium intake in humans, particularly when there are adequate levels of calcium, actually improves calcium utilization. All of this is why Doisy believes: "If calcium and magnesium intakes are high, or the balance between them is optimal, then there is a synergism between them such that both elements are better absorbed. Magnesium, for example, has a protective affect on the atherogenic score in rats only when the diet was high in calcium. Increasing the calcium content of animal diets, coupled with low magnesium intake, is detrimental to these animals. . , . I would like to advance the thesis that it is not only the absolute levels of magnesium that is important; the calcium-magnesium ratio should also be considered. That is, when the ratio is less than two to one, coronary heart disease and diabetes are less prevalent than when the ratio is higher."[11]

Direct evidence suggesting how important magnesium is in protecting us from cardiovascular heart disease is offered by reputable scientific studies. Examination of autopsy specimens from cattle that died from magnesium deficiencies clearly indicates obvious cardiovascular degeneration.[12] Heggtveit discovered a decreased magnesium content in the left ventricle of infarcted hearts compared to control hearts in sudden traumatic deaths.[13] Laurendeau also has seen a lower level of magnesium in the hearts of patients with myocardial necrosis, and this was more marked in diabetic subjects.[14] Animal studies clearly show that the amounts of fat deposits around the hearts of rats could be markedly reduced by the simple addition of magnesium.[15] In other studies it was also noted that this beneficial effect of magnesium lowering lipid levels was true only if adequate levels of calcium were also present. This, of course, confirms Doisy's position that calcium-magnesium ratios are extremely important, especially when dealing with cholesterol, cardiovascular disease and diabetes. We could continue with a listing of other numerous studies, all suggesting that magnesium is extremely important in maintaining cardiovascular integrity and health. But that is not the purpose of this chapter. Rather, it is important for the reader to understand that the mineral magnesium, like calcium or chromium, is just one more biochemical team player which must be present in order for us humans to resist the onslaughts of degenerative disease.

Granted then that an optimum intake of magnesium and calcium is important. The question remains whether the American diet contains adequate amounts of these nutrients. Unfortunately, according to scientific information, it does not! According to a study done by Schroeder[16] the average intake of magnesium in specific American hospitals averaged only 198 mg to 222 mg per day, a far cry from the 350 mg per day needed by the average 70 kg man. Schroeder also indicates that over one third of the average American diet contains calories derived from processed sugar and fat, both of which are almost entirely devoid of adequate magnesium and calcium levels. An individual eating such a diet receives approximately 120 mg of magnesium. On the other hand, if that same individual would reduce his fat and sugar intake, and simultaneously increase to whole cereal grains, and vegetables, fruits and nuts in his diet, his magnesium intake would soar to approximately 600 mg per day.

Another important point to remember when considering your daily mineral intake is the fact that there is a direct correlation between the amount of protein you eat and the loss or excretion of minerals in the human body. According to Nathan Pritikin, this correlation is a fact based on numerous scientific studies. Writes Pritikin:

There is a direct correlation between protein intake and excretion of minerals in humans. Margen has been testing this concept since 1965 with over two thousand University of California at Berkeley students. Findings on calcium are revealing: Increasing protein intake from 0 to 90 grams of nitrogen per day results in 800 percent of increase in calcium excretion, regardless of the calcium intake, which varied from 100 mg to 2300 mg per day. This effect was noted without exception in all studies conducted and was also repeated with synthetic amino acid mixtures.

Confirming studies on mineral loss through high protein, low carbohydrate diets come out of Fairleigh Dickinson University, where Dr. Carlton Fredericks has taught. Dr. Yacowitz found significant excretion losses in calcium, phosphorus, iron and zinc, as well as increased magnesium losses. . . . These studies may help us to understand why Western populations on high protein diets require so many mineral supplements, while underdeveloped populations like the Bantus on a 10 percent mostly vegetable intake require no supplements. On the average calcium intake of 350 mg per day, Walker reports that Bantu mothers give birth to an average of nine children and yet their bones and teeth do not show loss of density.[17]

Ironically, the twentieth century American diet is one seemingly designed for the intake of as little magnesium and calcium as is possible. Couple our dangerously high consumption of sugars and fats—all of which contain naked calories as far as vitamins and minerals are concerned—with our high animal protein intake, which according to scientific evidence accelerates mineral losses, and you have a situation in which magnesium and calcium, as well as other minerals, become extremely deficient. Such an environment sets the stage, as we have already seen, for the development of the number one killer in American culture: cardiovascular heart disease.

A very significant fact of cardiovascular disease is the relationship existing between hypertension (high blood pressure) and the grim statistic that over 15 percent of the deaths in this country can be directly attributed to it. It is a well-known idea that specific foods or chemicals can cause severe fluctuations in normal blood pressure. Allergic or otherwise maladaptive reactions to specific substances not only play an important role in determining blood sugar levels, as we have already seen, but also can determine particular blood pressure levels. Moreover, the relationship between the intake of large amounts of sodium (salt) and high blood pressure has been studied extensively, and since the average American diet consists of 10 grams of salt a day, and some contain much more, the importance of sodium as a causative agent in hypertension cannot be overlooked. Meneely and Ball for example, clearly demonstrated, as far back as 1958, that animals can be made severely hypertensive simply by feeding them large amounts of sodium chloride.[18] Numerous other studies since then have all confirmed their empirical findings. More recent studies, however, point to an even more disturbing possibility when considering the harmful effects of too much salt in the diet. In 1968, Dahl and his colleagues observed a phenomenon of what they called "post salt hypertension" which "could occur in man."[19] They discovered that when weanling rats were given 8 percent salt for only seven weeks, and then fed an ordinary rat chow containing less than 1 percent salt for six months, many of these animals became hypertensive during the high salt feedings—as expected—but almost one third of them, to these researchers' surprise, continued to have severe hypertension indefinitely. Rats with such a "post salt hypertension" also had a high mortality rate while eating their regular rat chow. The significance of this for humans is open to speculation. If human babies were, for example, given baby food containing high salt levels, the question now arises, in the light of Dahl's findings, whether this high sodium intake might negatively affect some of these children's lives as they grow older. That is, could a high salt baby food of today be causing the future hypertensives of tomorrow?

Granted then that allergic or otherwise maladaptive

reactions to specific foods and chemicals as well as the high intake of salt (sodium chloride) can directly cause hypertension, the question remains as to whether there are any other immediate causes of high blood pressure. The answer to this important question is in fact in the affirmative. Cadmium, a relatively unknown trace metal, has been directly linked to severe hypertension through experiments in which chronic feeding of very small doses of the trace element has resulted in elevated blood pressure and shortened survival. Schroeder gave rats drinking water containing only 0.0005 percent cadmium (i.e., 5 ppm) from weaning until death. Half of the rats fed cadmium became hypertensive at about eighteen months. None of his control animals became hypertensive. Writes Dr. Schroeder:

We have exposed rats for their lifetimes to small amounts, usually 5 ppm, of soluble metals in drinking water to find out whether we can reproduce in them human diseases. We have given 100 or more rats, half male and half female, vanadium, chromium, nickel, germanium, arsenic, selenium, zirconium, niobium, molybdenum, cadmium, tin, antimony, tellurium and lead. Only in those given cadmium was the full picture of human hypertension developed, with large hearts, changes in the blood vessels of the kidneys, high blood pressure, and an increase in atherosclerosis. Cadmium accumulates in both the human and the rat kidney, arteries, and liver, where it interferes with certain enzyme systems requiring zinc. Cadmium has more of an affinity for certain kidney tissues than does zinc, therefore displacing zinc and changing zinc-dependent reactions. It is also bound by blood vessels.

If we examine the ratio of zinc to cadmium in the American human kidney by weight, we find about 16 milligrams of zinc and over 11 milligrams of cadmium, or a ratio of 1.5. If we look at the primitive African kidney, the ratio is about 6. In the kidneys of beef the ratio is about 40 and pork 72. In the laboratory rat on a special low cadmium diet the ratio is 464–500 and in the mouse 451. In wild deer it was 23–70, in a coyote 54 and in a dog 24. In laboratory rats fed cadmium and having hypertension the average was 1.7 to less than 1.0. In people dying of hypertension the ratio was 1.4 to less than 1.0. Therefore, in mammals, there was much more cadmium in relation to zinc in Americans and in rats fed cadmium with hypertension than there was in any other mammal studied. The ratio of zinc to cadmium on the earth's crust is 500–1000. On these and many other studies, representing hundreds to thousands of analyses, we have come to the conclusion that cadmium in kidneys in relation to zinc is a contributing, if not sometimes the whole, cause of high blood pressure. In areas where the ratio is low the incidence of hypertension is high, and vice versa, based on the kidneys of 400 or more human subjects from around the world.

By injecting a special chelating agent, which binds cadmium more than it does zinc, we can remove some of the cadmium from rats' kidneys, replacing it with zinc. When we do this, we cure the hypertension overnight. If we continue to feed cadmium, hypertension slowly returns in several months, but can be cured again. This agent is under study in human subjects and shows promise.

Why does civilized man accumulate cadmium in his kidneys with age? The natural sources are food, water and air. If cadmium can displace zinc in his body, it is likely that food containing more than usual amounts of cadmium and less than usual amounts of zinc might slowly lead to the accumulation of cadmium. An excess of zinc would prevent accumulation of cadmium, a slight deficiency allow it. In table [X].1 are shown the amounts of zinc and cadmium in 250 common foods, and their ratios. Also in the table are a few representative foods with relatively large amounts of cadmium.[20]

Table [X].1

Average Concentrations of Zinc and Cadmium and their Ratios in Foods, ppm

Food	Zinc	Cadmium	Zinc/Cadmium
Seafood	17.5	0.79	22
Oysters	1280.0	3.40	378
Clams	27.8	0.58	48
Canned anchovies	17.7	5.39	3
Smoked kippers	20.3	1.28	16
Meats	30.6	0.88	35
Lamb chop	53.3	3.49	15
Chicken	29.0	2.0	15
Dairy Products	1.0	0.27	4
Butter	1.8	0.56	3

Food	Zinc	Cadmium	Zinc/Cadmium
Cereals and Grains	17.7	0.16	111
Gluten	48.5	0.51	97
Polished rice	1.6	0.06	27
Vegetables			
Legumes	10.7	0.03	357
Roots	3.4	0.07	49
Leaves and fruits	1.7	0.13	13
Oils and Fats	8.4	0.75	11
Olive oil	2.8	1.22	2
Margarine	1.6	0.8	2
Nuts	34.2	0.05	684
Fruits	0.5	0.04	13
Beverages	0.9	0.07	13
Average ratio			119
Whole human diet #1	6.1	0.19	32
diet #2	5.0	0.12	42
Purina Laboratory			
chow	58.1	0.63	92
Blue Spruce Farms			
rat chow	31.7	0.02	158
Grain			
Wheat	31.5	0.26	121
Farina	6.6	0.27	24
Patent Flour	6.4	0.38	17
First Clear Flour	15.9	0.26	61
Low Grade Flour	33.6	0.26	129
Red Dog	105.3	0.28	376
Shorts	106.0	0.92	115
Bran	100.2	0.88	113
Germ	133.4	1.11	120
Bread, whole wheat	5.3	0.15	35
Bread, white	1.2	0.22	5
Rye, whole	32.5	0.01	325
Wheat, gluten	48.5	0.51	97
Rye, oil	6.9	0.07	98
Oats	33.5	0.19	177
Barley	4.4	0.09	49
Buckwheat	25.5	0.27	95
Corn	3.8	0.12	32
Rice, American, polished	0.6	0.04	15
Rice, Japanese, polished	1.6	0.06	27
Sugars			
Sugar Cane	1.0	0.04	25
Granulated	1.3	0.06	22
Lump	0.2	0.27	<1
Molasses, household	2.9	0.56	3
", refining	3.3	0.83	4
", black strap	8.3	0.86	10

Food	Zinc	Cadmium	Zinc/Cadmium
Honey, refined	1.0	0.74	1
Fats			
Olive oil	2.8	1.22	2
Lard	0.5	0.05	10
Margarine	1.6	0.80	2
Butter	1.8	0.56	3
Beverage			
Coffee			
Infusion	0.03	0.006	5
" , dried	0.27	0.37	<1
Instant	0.10	0.006	16
" , dried	2.63	2.27	1
" , ground	3.10	0.32	10
Average			6
Caffeine-free			
Infusion 1	0.02	0.009	2
" 2	0.04	0.015	3
" 3	0.12	0.004	30
" 4	0.13	0.011	12
Dry 1	5.31	1.39	4
2	5.68	0.67	8
3	3.64	2.05	2
4	1.39	0.65	2
Average			8
Tea			
Infusion 1	0.33	0.01	33
" 2	0.24	0.006	40
" dried	0.44	0.56	<1
Black, leaves	34.36	1.61	21
Green, leaves, Japanese	36.30	2.50	11
infusion	0.04	0.001	40
Instant	0.20	0.008	25
" dry	8.00	1.38	6
Average			29
Cocoa, dry	48.65	0.67	73
Orange juice	0.65	0.01	65
Grape juice	3.11	0.07	44
Wines	1.41	0.085	17
Beers	0.33	0.01	33
Whiskey and gin	0.09	0.065	1

Obviously, the role of cadmium truly is a significant factor in producing hypertension. What is even more interesting, however, is the fact that, according to Dr. Schroeder, when cadmium is replaced with high levels of zinc, hypertension is "cured overnight." Parenthetically speaking, the

American propensity to refine their foods adds to the
cadmium-zinc ratio imbalance of which Dr. Schroeder
speaks. Refining of wheat and rice, for example, dramatically lowers the zinc levels, which leads to a correspondingly high cadmium-zinc ratio: refined flour is 1/26 cadmium-
zinc ratio by weight whereas wholewheat is 1/65 and
wheat is 1/120.

That zinc deficiency is involved as a causative factor
in vascular disease has been suggested by other well-known
researchers. Henzel (1971), for example, reported[21] that out
of twenty-four people placed on continued zinc supplementation of the diet for the treatment of arteriosclerosis,
eighteen of them showed distinct improvement. These
findings are further substantiated by Pidduck[22] who discovered that diabetics, who as we have seen have a very high
incidence of arteriosclerosis, actually excrete more zinc in
their urine than do normal subjects. Obviously, more conclu-
sive studies in this area of research need to be done, but
the evidence thus far clearly points to the fact that there is
indeed an actual relationship between the levels of cadmium in the blood, as well as plasma ratios of zinc to
cadmium, and the incidence of hypertension in the American general public.

Other minerals also have an important role in cardiovascular disease. Copper, in particular, like cadmium, is closely
linked to proper levels of zinc. Pansar has shown, for
example, that there is a positive correlation between high
levels of copper in the drinking water and the death rate
due to cardiovascular disease.[23] Moreover, another researcher
named Klevay has suggested a specific reason for Pansar's
statistical correlation of high copper levels and cardiovascular death rates. He observed that too little copper in
relation to zinc leads to an imbalance that may predispose
an individual to higher levels of cholesterol in the blood.
In 1973, Klevay empirically demonstrated that animals fed a
diet containing zinc and copper in a ratio of 17 to 1 had a
severely elevated cholesterol level compared to animals
receiving a diet with a ratio of 4 to 1.[24] Other researchers
have shown that there may be even more reasons for the

statistical correlation of high copper in cardiovascular disease. Morgan (1972)[25] has observed elevated serum copper levels in subjects dying from myocardial infarction. McKenzie and Kay have also demonstrated that individuals with hypertension excrete over 2.5 times more copper in their urine than do control groups with no hypertensive tendencies. Zinc levels in both groups were similar, which suggests that too much copper may be a causative factor in hypertension.[26] Again, more research needs to be done in this specific area of mineral imbalances, but there is enough evidence to date to strongly suggest a positive correlation between improper copper, cadmium, sodium and zinc plasma levels and the development of cardiovascular disease.

Some other minerals need at least a brief summary explanation of their actions in relation to diabetes and cardiovascular disease. Iron, a well-known mineral connected with anemia, is required by all humans, but has no known connection in the etiology of cardiovascular disease. However, there is a small segment of our population suffering from hemochromatosis. This particular disease is caused by an excess in iron storage and those who have it often have a form of diabetes called "bronze diabetes," in which the skin is discolored. Obviously any excessive intake of iron for those suffering from hemochromatosis is unquestionably contraindicated. In connection with diabetes, it is hypothesized that excessive iron storage might contribute to an induced chromium deficiency; that is, iron and chromium are chemically quite similar. If iron, for example, is in excess storage in the human body, chromium, which uses similar binding sites, might be crowded about, so to speak, especially since it is a trace element measured in much smaller quantities than is iron. One researcher, aware of this possibility, gave a subject suffering from hemochromatosis and diabetes small amounts of chromium. After the experimental chromium supplementation was administered, the patient's irregular glucose tolerance was normalized.[27] Obviously, the cure of one single patient does not prove anything, but it does open the door for those curious enough to research the matter in a more in-depth and scientifically controlled manner.

Recent interest has been given to the relationship existing between the administration of the trace element vanadium and the bile synthesis of cholesterol. A researcher named Mountain discovered decreased cholesterol levels and increased cholesterol catabolism (i.e., the process in which complex substances like cholesterol are converted into simpler substances, usually with an accompanying release of energy) in healthy subjects fed vanadium salts.[28]

Silicon is another trace element that needs to be researched in a more in-depth fashion. Next to oxygen, silicon is the most abundant element on earth. Loeper has reported that the silicon content of the human aorta decreases dramatically with age and that, even more interestingly, the artery of an individual suffering from arteriosclerosis contains severely decreased amounts of silicon.[29] Additional studies concerning silicon deficiencies should be done on more controlled subjects so as to confirm Loeper's findings.

The trace element lithium has been used by many psychiatrists for years in the treatment of depression and other disorders in mentally and emotionally ill patients. Van der Velde has observed that when treating such patients with lithium, there is a definite improvement in their glucose tolerance levels, which before the treatment were impaired.[30] Likewise, in an experiment with rats, Bhattacharya empirically observed an "insulin-like" effect of lithium on the glucose uptake in rats.[31]

In the 1980s, the time is ripe for physicians to become less concerned about the symptomatic drug treatment of disease and more interested in understanding the proper cellular-nutritional environment needed for optimum health. There is a need to examine interactions, antagonisms and synergisms between minerals, trace elements, as well as vitamins, amino acids, enzymes and hormones and between all groups to construct a fundamental, orderly, and logical determination of each of our individual health patterns. In order to be called true scientists or physicians, we must begin to fully understand all these complicated interactions between nutrients, enzymes and hormones. Scientifically controlled studies, therefore, now can, and positively should, be undertaken to ascertain what effect optimum levels of these nutrients properly supplied to people has on the incidence and severity of human vascular disease and diabetes. In short, the evidence presented in this book commands each and every one of us to look more deeply into that vast field of human Bio-Ecologic Medicine.

REFERENCES

1. Kobayashi, I. 1957. Geographical relationship between chemical nature of river water and death rate from apoplexy. *Benchte d. Ohara* Landivertsch Biologi 11:12–21.

2. Schroeder, H. A. 1960. Relation between mortality from cardiovascular disease and treated water supplies. *JAMA* 172:1908.

3. Masironi, R. 1970. Cardiovascular mortality in relation to radioactivity and hardness of local water supplies. *Bulletin WHO* 43:687.

4. Groover, M. E. and Antell, G. E. January 1972. Death rates following a sudden change in hardness of drinking water. *Epidemiology Newsletter* (American Heart Association), p. 16.

5. Malkiel-Shapiro, B. 1956. Parenteral magnesium sulfate therapy in coronary heart disease. *Medical Proceedings* 2:455–461.

6. Parsons, R. S., Butler, T. C. and Sellars, E. P. 1961. The treatment of coronary artery disease with parenteral magnesium sulfate. *Medical Proceedings* 5:487–498.

7. Brown, S. E. 1963. Magnesium and cardiovascular disease. *British Medical Journal* 2:118.

8. Doisy, R. S. 1978. Minerals and trace elements. *Diabetes, Obesity and Vascular Disease.* New York: Hemisphere, chap. 17, pp. 575–613.

9. Yacowitz, H., Fleischman, A. I. and Bierenbaum, M. L. 1965. Effects of oral calcium upon serum lipid in man. *British Medical Journal* 4:1352–1354.

10. Hendrix, D. M., Alcock, N. W. and Archibald, R. M. 1963. Competition between calcium, strontium, and magnesium for absorption in the isolated rat intestine. *Clinical Chemistry* 9:734–744.

11. Doisy, R. J. Minerals and trace elements, chap. 17, pp. 586, 594.

12. Duncan, C. W., Huffman, C. F. and Robinson, C. S. 1935. Magnesium studies in calves. Tetany produced by a ratio of milk or milk with various supplements. *Journal of Biological Chemistry* 108:35–44.

13. Heggtveit, H. A., Tanser, P. and Hunt, B. 1969. Magnesium contents of normal and ischemic human hearts. *International Congress of Clinical Pathology* 7:53.

14. Laurendeau, E., and Duriusseau, J. P. 1963. Electrolytes in aging human and animal normal and pathological hearts. *Members 55th Congress Mundial Cardiol* 5:245.

15. Vitale, J. J.; Hellerstein, E. E.; Hegsted, D. M.; Nakamura, M.; and Farkman, A. 1959. Dietary magnesium and calcium in atherogenesis and renal lesions. *American Journal of Clinical Nutrition* 7:13–22.

16. Schroeder, H. A., Nason, A. P. and Tipton, I. H. 1969. Essential metals in man: magnesium. *Journal of Chronic Diseases* 21:815–841.

17. Pritikin, Nathan. 1976. High carbohydrate diets: maligned and misunderstood. *Journal of Applied Nutrition* 28(3 & 4): 63–64.

18. Meneely, G. R. 1958. Experimental epidemiology of chronic sodium chloride toxicity. *American Journal of Medicine* 25:713.

19. Dahl, L. K. 1968. Effects of chronic excess salt ingestion. *Civic Resources* 22:11.

20. Schroeder, H. A. 1973. *The Trace Elements and Man*, Old Greenwich, CT: Devin-Adair Company, pp. 98–99.

21. Henzel, J. H.; Keitzer, F. W.; Lichti, L. L.; and DeWeese, M. 1971. Efficacy of zinc medication as a therapeutic modality in atherosclerosis. *Trace Substances in Environmental Health.* ed. D. D. Hemphill. Columbia: University of Missouri, vol. 4, pp. 336–341.

22. Pidduck, H. G., Wren, P. J. and Price, Evans. 1970. Hyperzincuria of Diabetes Mellitus. *Diabetes* 19:240–247.

23. Pansar, S. et al. 1975. Coronary heart disease and drinking water. *Journal of Chronic Diseases* 28:259–287.

24. Klevay, L. M. 1973. Decreased copper in human food since 1942. *Federation Proceedings* 35(3):342 (abstract).

25. Morgan, J. M. 1972 b. Tissue copper and lead content in ischemic heart disease. *Archives of Environmental Health* 25:26–28.

26. McKenzie, M. M. Urinary excretion of cadmium, zinc and copper in hypertensive women. *New Zealand Medical Journal* 80:68–70.

27. Levine, R. A. Effects of oral chromium supplementation on the glucose tolerance of elderly human subjects. *Metabolism* 17:114–125.

28. Mountain, S. T., Stockell, F. R. and Stokinger, H. L. 1956. Effect of ingested vanadium on cholesterol and phospholipid metabolism in the rabbit. *Proceedings of the Society to Explore Biological Medicine* 92:582–587.

29. Loeper, J., Loeper, J. and Lemaire, A. 1966. Etude du cilcium en biologie et au course de l'atherome. *Presse Med* 74:865–868.

30. Van der Velde, C. D. and Gordon, M. W. 1969. Manic depressive illness diabetes mellitus, and lithium carbonate. *Archives of General Psychiatry* 21:478–485.

31. Bhattacharya, G. 1964. Influence of lithium on glucose metabolism in rats and rabbits. *Archives of Biochemistry and Biophysics. Acta* 93:644–646.

CHAPTER ELEVEN

EPA, GLA and prostaglandins:
A potential breakthrough
in the prevention and
treatment of cardiovascular disease

Not since the days when insulin and cortisone were discovered has there been so much interest in a group of therapeutic chemicals normally found in the human body. Scientists calculate that since the beginning of the 1980s, over two hundred research papers are being published every month on a new group of very important chemicals produced by the body. These chemicals are known as prostaglandins. They were not always so celebrated because at the time of their discovery, over fifty years ago, there were very few sophisticated methods by which they could be scientifically studied. Now all that has changed.

Prostaglandins are hormonelike chemical substances which act as messengers which regulate vital metabolic processes throughout the body. Obviously, since scientists have only recently begun to investigate them seriously, there is much more to be learned. To date, there are about thirty known prostaglandins; they are divided into three major categories based on their number of chemical double bonds: series one, two and three. The immediate effect of prostaglandins is on the same organ or tissue that produces them. Their effect is usually very brief—yet very powerful—because they are not stored and are quickly inactivated by specific enzymes. Interestingly, almost every tissue of the body produces prostaglandins; yet the same prostaglandin may have various functions in different tissues. All of this is why scientists agree that prostaglandins are a very interesting group of chemicals for which a great deal more clinical research needs to be done.

But what does all this discussion about prostaglandins have to do with arteriosclerosis? The answer to this important question lies in a thorough understanding of the scientific evidence concerning plasma lipid and triglyceride levels in Greenlandic Eskimos. As far back as 1926, it was reported in the *Journal of the American Medical Association* that 142 Eskimo adults between the ages of forty and sixty were medically examined and found to be completely free of any signs of cardiovascular disease.[1] These findings are in total agreement with other scientific studies done on Greenlandic Eskimos.[2] As we have previously discussed, Roger J. Williams, Ph.D., of the Clayton Foundation, believes that since adults of widely different ethnic stock can physically thrive, without any cardiovascular symptom formation, on a high fat, high cholesterol, high caloric diet, "the evidence points strongly [contrary to popular medical thinking] toward the conclusion that the nutritional microenvironment of the body cells—involving minerals, amino acids, and vitamins—is crucial, and that the amount of fat or cholesterol consumed is relatively inconsequential."[3] As clinical studies have clearly demonstrated, vitamin B6, which is abundantly present in the raw liver consumed by the Eskimos, is but one nutrient extremely important in this regard.[4] Indeed, as we have seen in the preceding chapters, minerals, amino acids, fiber, as well as other vitamins—and all their corresponding nutrient ratios—are crucial when attempting to maintain cardiovascular cellular integrity. But in addition to these nutrient ratios, new scientific evidence is pointing to another important biochemical link in the chain of cardiovascular health. We have in mind those all-important prostaglandins and eicosapentaenoic acid (EPA).

According to a recently published article in the well-respected scientific journal Lancet, the incidence of atherosclerotic heart disease, including coronary arterial disease, in Greenlandic Eskimos is extremely low.[5] From 1963 to 1967, only three cases of these diseases were reported in the Eskimo population of Greenland. Moreover, not a single established case of diabetes mellitus is known to have been reported in the population of the Greenlandic Uhanak district. Since diabetes mellitus and atherosclerotic heart disease afflict literally millions of suffering Americans in the 1980s, these statistical figures have attracted the serious attention of many scientists throughout our nation.[6]

The word "Eskimo" is of Red Indian Origin and means "people eating raw meat." The food of the Greenlandic Eskimos still living as hunters and/or fishermen consists predominantly of meat from whales, seals, sea birds and fish (usually halibut and salmon). Needless to say, their food is extremely rich in protein and fat, and poor in carbohydrates. Green leafy vegetables, potatoes, squash, spinach and the like are seldom eaten by these healthy-hearted people living in a world surrounded by ice, snow and bone-freezing temperatures.

Doctors have been saying for years that large amounts of fat in the diet are strongly correlated with coronary heart disease. Why, therefore, you might ask, can a group of people who consume such large amounts of protein and fat have such a low incidence of atherosclerotic heart disease? If you are concerned about this seemingly confusing correlation, you are not alone. Scientific researchers have, until recently, also been baffled by these curious facts, but based on new statistical as well as clinical evidence, they now believe that there is a logical explanation. The new link in their chain of total understanding centers around a tongue-twisting fatty EicosaPentaenoic Acid (commonly referred to as EPA). EPA is a direct precursor of the important prostaglandin PGE_3. There is a large amount of EPA in fish:

you get, for example, about 20 percent EPA in scallops, oysters, red caviar, mackerel, or by taking marine oils like cod liver oil.

One interesting fact about EPA came to light when the polyunsaturated fatty acids in the diet and the tissues of Eskimos eating their usual high fat and protein diet and of Danes in Copenhagen living on an American type diet were scientifically compared and studied. It was discovered that the longer chain polyunsaturated fatty acid EPA (C20:5w3) found in marine oils was present in much larger amounts in the Eskimos. In fact, EPA was present to the extent of 10 percent of the total plasma lipids (blood fats) in the Eskimos, whereas in the Danes, living on a diet especially low in marine fats, it was nearly absent. And, of course, the Danes had a much higher statistical record of coronary heart disease as compared to the Eskimos.[7]

Scientists are now beginning to understand the compli- cated reasons why this long chain polyunsaturated fatty acid called EPA is so beneficial in maintaining cardiovascular integrity. William E. Connor, M.D., for example, supported by a research grant from the National Heart, Lung and Blood Institute and the Division of Research Resources at the National Institute of Health, has offered very interest- ing evidence concerning the dietary intake of Omega-3 fatty acids, and in particular EPA and DHA (DocosaHexaenoic Acid, a major fatty acid of the brain and central nervous system). EPA, he suggests, is highly correlated to the Eskimos' extremely low incidence of coronary heart disease and strokes. Dr. Connor and his group of research scien- tists assessed the effects of different dietary fats (e.g., vegetable oil, and fish-marine oil) on blood lipids and platelet function in fourteen patients with hyperlipidemia (high blood fats). They discovered that when comparing the hypolipidemic (lowering blood fats) effects of Omega-3 marine oil and Omega-6 vegetable oils, both dietary fats actually lowered plasma cholesterol and triglyceride levels. However, the marine oil subjects' cholesterol fell a dra- matic 32 percent as compared to the vegetable oil subjects' less dramatic 19 percent. Similarly, the marine oil subjects' triglycerides plunged 66 percent as compared again to the vegetable oil subjects' 38 percent.[8] These results suggest that EPA containing marine oils have a very significant "hypolipidemic effect" in man. As such, they may prove to be an extremely useful natural substance powerful enough to normalize the all too often high cholesterol and triglyceride levels found in our modern American population.

In addition, Dr. Connor's team of specialists discovered to their surprise that Omega-3 fatty acids also had "anti-thrombotic properties."[9] What this means is that EPA is intimately involved in body processes that inhibit blood clots (obstructions to circulation) of the heart or blood vessels. Platelets are microscopic structures of the blood that play a very important role in blood coagulation and blood thrombus formation. When a small blood vessel is injured, platelets adhere to each other around the edges of the injury; they then form a "plug" that covers the injured area. The plug or blood clot formed soon retracts and stops the loss of blood. Without blood platelets, we could all literally bleed to death when injured.

However, when platelets in the blood become too "sticky," they can clump abnormally fast. It is thought that such rapid platelet aggregation contributes to cardiovascular (heart and blood vessel) disease. Excessive platelet clumping is known to be associated with eating too much sugar and not enough manganese. Processing, by the way, removes most of the manganese from sugar cane. Researchers are convinced, however, that EPA rich marine oils inhibit platelet aggregation and adhesion—thus their "anti-thrombotic" effect in the body.

Theoretically, EPA has two major physiological functions in the treatment of atherosclerosis. First, EPA displaces arachidonic acid in the platelets; this process inhibits the enzyme cyclooxygenase and, therefore, prevents the production of the aggregating or platelet clumping prostaglandin, thromboxane A_2. Second, EPA in the blood vessel wall has been shown to stimulate the synthesis of the very powerful prostaglandin, prostacyclin PGI_2.

Prostacyclin is a prostaglandin or hormonelike substance

which regulates vital metabolic processes throughout the body. To date, there are about thirty known prostaglandins; they are divided into three major categories based on their number of chemical double bonds: series one, two and three. Prostacyclin is a member of the two series prosta-glandins, and without question is the most potent protector against platelet clumping and blood vessel and bronchial constriction. In short, prostacyclin is a very important chemical in all the blood vessels and the lungs and is the major reason why our platelets keep circulating as they should. Thromboxane is another two series prostaglandin, but it is the most powerful platelet aggregator of the body. We obviously need platelet aggregation; without it, we would not be able to stop bleeding after sustaining an injury. The problem is in maintaining a proper balance between platelet aggregation and proper platelet circulation.

If there was a way to increase the prostacyclin in our body, without simultaneously raising the thromboxane lev-els, perhaps we Americans, like the Eskimos, could live a life free from the ravages of cardiovascular disease. Dr. Connor, professor of medicine, University of Oregon, has discovered that EPA in the diet is precisely that natural substance that can accomplish this task. For EPA—a stimulator of the potent prostaglandin, prostacyclin, and an inhibitor of the equally potent prostaglandin, thromboxane A_2—significantly lowered platelet aggregation in all of the fourteen individuals he tested.[10] And if there is less platelet aggregation, there is a reduced chance of forming the death dealing blood clots that so commonly occur in heart attacks, strokes or other cardiovascular related complications.

In short, many prominent researchers are finding that EPA not only lowers cholesterol and triglyceride levels, but it also is involved in preventing blood clots. As Dr. Connor puts it: "Our results suggest that the W-3 [Omega-3] fatty acids found in fish liver oils are both hypolipidemic and antithrombotic. With these two properties, W-3 [Omega-3] fatty acids may be useful in the prevention and treatment of atherosclerotic disease."[11]

Incidentally, if you are a smoker, there is more disturbing medical news for you to consider. Recent evidence suggests that nicotine inhibits prostacyclin production. Indirectly, therefore, smoking can lead to a greater likelihood of rapid platelet aggregation and adhesion. The results of this metabolic possibility are a greater potential for blood clots as well as cardiovascular degeneration and disease. A smoker could take more EPA rich marine oil as a potential preventive measure. But that would be like accelerating the gas pedal of your car (i.e., smoking) while simultaneously stepping on the brake (ingesting EPA). A better alternative would be to take optimum levels of marine oil, eat more EPA rich fish in your diet, and stop smoking!

A very interesting prostaglandin research study is currently being done by Dr. David Horrobin at the Institute for Innovative Medicine in Montreal. Dr. Horrobin believes that the "one" series prostaglandins are very essential in maintaining cardiovascular integrity. One of the most important of this particular series prostaglandins is PGE_1. "The level of PGE_1," writes Dr. Horrobin, "is of crucial importance to the body. A fall in the level of PGE_1 will lead to a potentially catastrophic series of untoward consequences including increased vascular reactivity, enhanced blood clotting, elevated cholesterol production, and diabetic-like changes in insulin release. . . ."[12] In short, PGE_1 has many varied beneficial effects in the body, but those most essentially related to cardiovascular health are: 1. it dilates blood vessels; 2. it lowers blood pressure; 3. it prevents platelet aggregation and adhesion; and 4. it inhibits cholesterol formation.

To insure that we have an optimum level of PGE_1 in our diet, we must eat liberal amounts of cis-linoleic acid. The metabolic pathway of this particular chemical is as follows: cis-linoleic acid is converted into gamma-linolenic acid (GLA); GLA is then converted into dihomo-gamma-linolenic acid (DGLA); DGLA is finally converted into PGE_1. It should be emphasized that cis-linoleic acid occurs in such cold pressed oils as safflower oil (73 percent), evening primrose oil (73 percent), corn oil (57 percent), sunflower oil (58 percent), soybean oil (51 percent), peanut oil (29 percent) and olive oil (8 percent).[13] Trans-linoleic acid, on the other hand, which is present in margarine, hydrogenated oils, and unfortunately in a dangerously large proportion of the American diet, actually blocks the proper utilization of cis-linoleic acid; it also simultaneously increases the need for more essential fatty acids found in the cold pressed oils previously mentioned.[14] Other factors which inhibit the proper conversion of cis-linoleic acid into GLA and PGE_1 are: 1. a diet rich in saturated fats; 2. moderate to high consumption of alcohol; 3. diabetes; 4. nutrient deficiencies such as zinc, magnesium and vitamin B6; and 5. viral infections, radiation, old age and cancer.

It is important to understand that cis-linoleic acid occurs in nature's foods, whereas trans-linoleic acid—with very few exceptions—is a product of man-made or processed foods. Please bear in mind that natural vegetable oils contain large amounts of cis-linoleic acid, but commercial processing of these oils aimed at improving their stability, odor and shelf life converts a significant amount of the beneficial cis-linoleic acid to the more unhealthy form, trans-linoleic acid. All of this discussion emphasizes the sad but true fact that the American diet, with all of its margarines and processed salad oils, is tragically blocking the proper utilization of those factors which significantly prevent cardiovascular complications from occurring.

Even though many aspects of the American lifestyle inhibit the proper conversion of cis-linoleic acid into GLA and PGE_1, there is one substance that contains beneficial levels of concentrated GLA. This substance is the seed oil of a plant known as the evening primrose. This plant originated in the eastern United States and was extensively used by the American Indian for medicinal purposes. The wild evening primrose has now been domesticated and its oil contains approximately 9 percent by weight of GLA. The remaining part of the oil is very similar to raw safflower or sunflower oil, containing approximately 73 percent of cis-linoleic acid. Primrose oil is of particular interest because it alone contains initially a significant percentage of

GLA. GLA, of course, with the aid of optimum levels of vitamin B6, is rapidly converted into DGLA. Likewise, DGLA, in combination with vitamins C and B3, is then converted into that all important cardiovascular-related prostaglandin known as PGE_1.

As with any chemical within the human body, whether it is a vitamin, mineral, enzyme, amino acid or essential fatty acid, specific biochemical need levels of each substance must be determined on a biochemically individual basis. This idea, of course, implies that when using these substances in the treatment of illness, one should always keep in mind that what helps one individual in his progression toward optimum health may not do so for another. Specific nutrient needs may vary a thousandfold among individuals. Therefore, an individually determined treatment program using any natural chemical substance normally found in the body should be the plan of action. Such a program will preferably include analysis and subsequent treatment based on clinically demonstrated deficiencies.

Moreover, we must always keep in mind that no one specific chemical within the human body, such as vitamin A, calcium, tyrosine, EPA, GLA or PGE_1, cures anything by itself. For these chemicals, and many more just like them, are always team players. That is, they work together for the benefit of the whole body. Sometimes when you increase the level of one of these chemicals, you need more of another. A dietary increase of highly unsaturated and essential fatty acids, for example, like EPA in marine oils, might raise your need levels for vitamin E. Other nutrient interactions still unknown at this time might also be important. Therefore, research must in the future always take into account all the specific interactions of all the various chemicals normally occurring in the human body before any scientific conclusions can be considered as final or absolute.

REFERENCES

1. Lieb, C. July 1926. Health of a carnivorous race. May 1927. *JAMA*.

2. Dyerberg, J. June 1971. Plasma lipid and lipoprotein pattern in Greenlandic west-coast Eskimos. *Lancet*, pp. 1143–1145.

3. Williams, R. J. 1973. *Nutrition Against Disease*. New York: Bantam Books, p. 249.

4. Rinehart, J. F. 1949. Arteriosclerotic lesions in pyridoxine-deficient monkeys. *American Journal of Pathology* 25:481–491; McCully, K. S. July 1969. Vascular pathology of homocysteinemia. *American Journal of Pathology* 56:111–128.

5. Thorngren, M. November 28, 1981. Effects of an 11-week increase in dietary EPA on bleeding time, lipids, and platelet aggregation. *Lancet*, p. 1190.

6. Bang, H. O. 1972. Plasma lipids in Greenlandic west coast Eskimos. *Acta. Med. Scand.* 192:85.

7. Kronmann, N. 1980. Epidemiological studies in the Upernairk district of Greenland. Incidence of chronic disease. *Acta. Med. Scand.* 208:401–406.

8. Connor, W. E. Dietary fish oils, plasma lipids, and platelets in man. Research Grant HL-25687—to be published—from the National Heart, Lung and Blood Institute.

9. *Ibid*.

10. *Ibid*.

11. *Ibid*.

12. Horrobin, D. F. 1980. *Medical Hypothesis* 6:785–800.

13. *Dairy Council Digest*. November-December 1975, 46:6.

14. Passwater, R. A. 1981 *Evening Primrose Oil*. New Canaan, CT: Keats Publishing, Inc. p. 5.

CHAPTER TWELVE

The difficult role of change

Medical education as it is today is basically lacking an orientation in Bio-Ecologic Medicine. To many physicians, though well trained in established values and techniques, the applications of Bio-Ecologic Medicine remain a mystery, and therefore, to them, the physicians using these new applications in their medical practice remain equally mysterious.

The science of diabetology is fraught with dogmatic schools of thought which undoubtedly stem from the uncertainties of knowledge about the difficulties in treating this disease. Obviously, this dogmatic atmosphere of thought creates a communication problem for any new formula or fact. With this in mind, we do not anticipate a ready acceptance of our observations concerning the degree of reversibility of the chemical and clinical stages of diabetes mellitus by ecologic-metabolic diagnosis and treatment. Each physician will have to see the evidence for himself. However, the results of ecologic-metabolic diagnosis and treatment of diabetes have been sufficiently rewarding for us to risk sharing our observations with our fellow physicians as well as laymen.

Criticism, no matter what its motivation, is eventually profitable since it forces those maintaining the new formulation to develop maximum justification for its existence. It seems evident that when subjects with many unknowns, such as religion, philosophy, the cause of schizophrenia, the cause of diabetes and so forth are dealt with, many schools of thought emerge for reasons of anxiety reduction. These belief systems develop tenacious followers who are like politico-religious zealots ready to defend their cause to the death. Such a rigid attitude mediates against incorporating new and especially contrary information into the belief system. Indeed, we are asking for a lot of change of frequently held and sometimes cherished beliefs when we propose from our empirically received evidence that the varying stages of the diabetes disease process, including the usual chemical diabetes phase observed in millions of people, can be understood as a decipherable response to isolable environmental substances and that monitoring the patient's biochemistry during and after these reactions provides valuable guidelines as to cause and treatment.

Hypotheses are a necessary aspect for progress. Hypotheses have the chance of being sufficiently sound to contribute to progress. The formulator may, by chance, be judged as way ahead, as well as running the risk of being judged as way out, or worse. Even if and when correct, formulations from basic science are likely to have a twenty-year wait before practical clinical application occurs due to the natural resistance to change stemming from an assortment of personal, social and economic factors.[1] We have dared to share our formulations for which we believe we have objectively observed a usefulness in our patients. We hope the reader will be generous enough to allow the right of formulation, even though all the answers are not yet in.

Thomas S. Kuhn[2] has become well known for his "Structure of Scientific Revolution." The following quotation summarizes his observations: "The invention of other new theories regularly and appropriately evokes the same response from some of the specialists on whose area of special competence they impinge. For these men the new theory implies a change in the rules governing the prior practice of normal science. Inevitably therefore it reflects upon much scientific work they have already successfully completed. That is why a new theory however special its range of application is seldom or never just an increment to what is already known. Its stimulation requires the reconstruction of prior theory and the reevaluation of prior fact, an intrinsically revolutionary process that is seldom completed by a single man and never overnight."

Generally speaking, doctors theoretically believe that the disease process should be rationally treated as a disease state. However, in clinical practice physicians often ignore the disease process and resort to symptomatic treatment. We hope that the evidences presented in this book will awaken those fine qualities doctors potentially have and not only encourage a rational therapeutic approach to the basic diabetes disease process but also simultaneously discourage the approach which attempts to offer only a palliative relief of the diabetic's symptoms. This is the only way we can serve our patients best in preventing and/or reversing their steadily encroaching degenerative diseases, whether these are expressed as mental or physical diseases.

REFERENCES

1. Ferguson, M. 1980. *The Aquarian Conspiracy*. Los Angeles: J. P. Tarcher.

2. Kuhn, T.S. 1970. *The Structure of Scientific Revolution*. Chicago: University Chicago Press.

A physician's guide to a bio-ecologic examination and subsequent treatment

Bio-ecologic examination

A Bio-Ecologic examination has special value in determining the nature of both physical and mental degenerative diseases. Since the diabetes mellitus disease process is central to many degenerative diseases, it is especially important to understand the fundamental aspects of such an examination. These central component parts of the bio-ecologic examination are:

1. History and initial examination.

2. One and preferably two stress days with associated laboratory examinations.

3. Five days of avoidance of commonly used foods and frequently contacted chemicals.

4. Deliberate provocative exposure testing with monitoring for symptoms and blood sugar changes.

5. Intradermal or sublingual serial dilution testing of specific items.

6. Inhalation testing.
7. Cytotoxic testing.
8. Total IgE and RAST.
9. Phenolic food compound testing.

1. HISTORY AND INITIAL EXAMINATION

First, a medical assessment of the patient's chief complaint and prior medical history is performed. There should be special attention given to gestation and infancy and how they relate to food and chemical exposure and possible maladaptive reactions. Second, an assessment is made of possible addictions to coffee, tobacco, alcohol, marijuana or other street drugs. Food binges are analyzed, and the frequency with which each food is eaten is analyzed. The degree of exposure to various chemicals at home and work is considered. Mental status and motor function are observed. Blood pressure, pulse, reflexes and gait are studied. Medications in current use are evaluated. Based on the evidence collected from all of the above, an initial impression is made. A formulation is then made and an initial recommendation is offered.

2. STRESS DAYS

During these two days, the patient continues to use frequently eaten foods while a laboratory assessment is being made of his or her biological state. On the first stress day, the patient is instructed to eat, among other things, a big serving of such lysine-bearing foods as either fish, turkey, chicken or pork. A twenty-four hour urine is collected during this day and sent to the specialty reference lab for a complete amino acid profile. Such a profile consists of thirty-nine amino acids plus carnosine and anserine analyzed by chromatography. The second day also involves a collection of a twenty-four hour urine sample and a repeat of the amino acid profile. Breakfast on this day consists of lactose for a lactose tolerance test. During the rest of the day, the patient eats especially high protein foods but also includes a wide assortment of his or her commonly used foods. High carnosine foods are to be eaten this day such as beef, pork, rabbit and salmon; as well as the anserine foods chicken, turkey and duck. On the morning after the first stress day, blood samples are drawn for insulin, complete blood count and a parathyroid profile, if the patient has complained of weakness or feeling worse with exercise. A broad spectrum chemistry screen analysis should also be done at this time. It includes alkaline phosphatase, gamma glutamyl transferase, LDH, SGOT, SGPT, glucose, triglycerides, cholesterol, sodium, potassium, chloride, CO_2 content, calcium, inorganic phosphorus, uric acid, urea nitrogen, creatinine, total protein, albumin, globulin, A/G ratio, bun/creatinine, anion gap, osmolality, calcium (ionized) and total bilirubin. Glycohemoglobin and cholyglycine (gall bladder test) are also run.

The twenty-four hour urine of the second day is studied for:

1. Spillage of reducing sugar (galactose).

2. Thirty-nine amino acids, carnosine and anserine.

3. Kynurenic and xanthurenic acid spillage for B6 function test.

4. Formiminoglution acid spillage (FIGLU test) for folic acid function.

A blood and serum sample is drawn and sent to a specialty lab for a paramecium study. This test assesses the blood level of B12, folic acid, B6, thiamin, niacin, biotin, riboflavin, pantothenic acid, vitamin A, vitamin C, vitamin E and beta-carotene. Within the first two days, a hair test biopsy is run. During the second stress day, the patient receives 5 grams of tryptophan, 3 grams of methionine and 10 grams of histidine. The tryptophan is used to stress B6, the histidine is used to stress folic acid; the methionine is used to stress methionine metabolism, the disorder of which is characteristic of addiction. A celiac test is done on the second stress day and the day after Stress II or on separate days when blood can be drawn in A.M. after all night fast and alkaline phosphatase test is done. An all day stress of wheat, rye, barley and buckwheat test meals are given followed by a repeat alkaline phosphatase test the following morning. A 20 percent drop in alkaline phosphatase gives evidence of celiac disease (gluten enteropathy).

The above tests have been the routine for a sizable number of patients. Recently we have changed to a set of more functional tests. These consist of blood tests for:

Erythrocyte glutathione peroxidase (status for selenium).
Erythrocyte glutathione reductase (status for B2).
Erythrocyte transketolase for thiamine nutritional status.
Monoamine oxidase in platelets.

The twenty-four hour urine test includes: methyl-malonic acid for B12 function, dopamine, norephinephrine, 3-methoxy-4-hydroxy phenly glycol and in some cases a kryptopyrrole test.

Also the immunology studies have been changed to consist of a protein profile (quantitative):
Albumin
Alpha-1-acid glycoprotein
Alpha-1-antitrypsin
Alpha-2-macroglobulin
C3 complement
C4 complement
Haptoglobin
IgA
IgG
IgM
Low density lipoprotein
Transferrin

A phospholipid fatty acid profile is done consisting of sixteen essential fats, Serum C-reactive protein and T&B lymphocytes.

Within the first two days a hair sample is taken, approximately 5 grams or 1 tablespoonful of hair clipped from the nape of the neck area. The hair is clipped as closely to the neck as possible and is no more than two inches in length. This sample is sent a specialty laboratory for a mineral hair analysis.

3. FIVE DAY AVOIDANCE PERIOD

The five day period of avoidance can be either a fast on nonchemically treated water only or a period of eating uncommonly used foods as test meals. The goal of this procedure is to avoid commonly used foods and frequently contacted chemicals for a sufficient time period for metabolic recovery from the state of addiction to occur. It usually requires about five days. The first three days are the more serious symptom evoking days of withdrawal from the state of addiction.

During this time, the saliva pH is monitored with pHydrion paper using a double cartridge with a range of 6–8 on one side and 5.7–6.2 on the other side. The normal reading for saliva pH ranges from 6.4 to 6.8. In diabetics, the saliva and urine pH (abnormal below 6) is taken every four hours day and night. If an abnormality is found in either reading, then one teaspoon of sodium-potassium bicarbonate (ratio 2:1) is given. The pH is again taken in two hours. If this does not properly control the pH, then intravenous sodium bicarbonate is administered: 75 mEq as the adult dose.

In the late afternoon of the first three to five days of avoidance, the following are administered intravenously over a thirty minute or more period combined in 100 cc .9 percent sodium chloride: 12½ grams of sodium ascorbate, 1000 mg B6, 100 mg B3 as niacinamide, 1250 mg B5 as pantothenol, calcium phosphorus containing 250 mg of calcium, magnesium chloride containing 2 grams of magnesium and 5000 units Heparin. This combination of nutrients does much to allay withdrawal symptoms and maintain a reasonable chemical metabolic homeostasis during the withdrawal phase of addiction.

A. In nutritionally debilitated cases, intravenous amino acids, intravenous lipids or intravenous total nutrition may be used with the addition of vitamin C, B6, B5, B3, calcium phosphorus, magnesium and Heparin.

B. Due to a particularly unstable acid base balance, even nondiabetic infants and children should be considered as acidosis prone. Be ready to give intravenous sodium bicarbonate in case of weakness, lethargy or a sustained drop in saliva or urine pH. The dose is dependent on body weight. The adult dose for sodium bicarbonate intravenously is 75 mEq. Be sure to maintain adequate fluid intake. Adult fluid intake is based on ten glasses of water per twenty-four hours. Infants and children should be judged on percentage of body weight.

C. Seizure cases require special attention. Minor seizures, however, pose no special problem. In these cases, antiseizure medication can be gradually decreased over a minimum of five days while monitoring IV nutrition or decreased more slowly over a two week period. With grand mal seizures, on the other hand, the following considerations need to be made:

1. Antiseizure medication should be monitored during avoidance period and provocative testing period.

2. Educate the responsible adult in the mechanics of caring for the patient during a seizure.

3. Provide a tank of oxygen. Also give a positive pressure breathing bag, mask and a rubber mouthpiece containing a breathing hole for the patient's home use.

4. In the more severe cases, do cytotoxic testing, RAST testing and serial dilution intradermal testing before starting the five day avoidance. Later, provocative testing should be done to determine the value of avoidance of foods and chemicals incriminated by these tests. Some highly reactive foods on the cytotoxic study need not be included in the provocative testing. However, many seizure cases electing to have a bio-ecologic diagnosis and treatment have multiple uncontrolled seizures.

5. Be prepared to stop status epilepticus with intravenous medication: phenobarbital or Dilantin. I [W.P.] have never observed a case of status epilepticus evoked by food and chemical testing. One case of status epilepticus requiring intravenous

medication was inadvertently evoked by a chance exposure to petrochemical hydrocarbons. The doctor electing to diagnose and treat epileptics must be prepared for all eventualities.

D. Asthmatics should have bronchial dilators and oxygen available. Graduate down the oral medication and be ready to return to it. If necessary, proceed with provocative testing while on medication.

E. Those on steroids other than Addison's cases can usually be graduated down over the five day period. Be ready to reinstate the steroids if necessary. If need be, proceed with provocative testing while on the steroids.

F. Nonacidosis prone, noninsulin dependent diabetics pose no special problem other than the necessity of frequent monitoring of blood sugar, saliva and urine pH. Keeping the acid base balance normal with sodium-potassium alkali salts is also important. Those who have been judged as insulin dependent juvenile diabetics and acidosis prone insulin dependent maturity-onset diabetics are monitored as described above. However, they are never fasted and their insulin is continued as usual using essentially the same criteria as they are accustomed to for determining their insulin requirement. Using the micromethod of blood glucose determination, the blood glucose is determined before and after each meal and every four hours (even at night) when not eating. If the A.M. blood sugar is normal (110 to 115 mg percent or less), the first test meal is given without insulin. Insulin is given when a test meal does not return to normal in four hours. If there is no recovery after the first test meal, then usually a long acting insulin plus regular insulin is used. The patient keeps with him a readily available form of sugar and is instructed in its use in the event the blood sugar drops to below 60 mg percent. The sugar used is usually maple sugar or dates. Should this be necessary, the blood sugar is retested in one hour. From the A.M. fasting blood sugar, a judgment is made as to how much long acting and regular insulin is needed.

In juvenile-type insulin dependent diabetics, it is a wise plan to do cytotoxic and RAST testing. The frequently used foods that are negative on these tests are then tested by serial dilution intradermal testing. If the case is in poor control, the option may be to first remove cytotoxic, RAST and intradermal positive foods even though these tests do not in themselves conclusively prove a direct relationship to disordered carbohydrate metabolism. In removing these test positive foods and chemicals from the diet, one must be prepared for a drastic reduction in insulin requirements. It has been my observation that, characteristically, insulin requirements will immediately be reduced by two thirds when test positive foods and chemicals are avoided. This is true of bona fide insulin dependent juvenile diabetics. One gains the impression that even though the primary cause of juvenile insulin dependent diabetes may not be ecologic in origin, a substantial mal-adaptive reactivity to environmental substances secondarily develops. Indeed, the insulin dependent diabetic needs Bio-Ecologic diagnosis and treatment as much as the completely reversible noninsulin dependent diabetic.

4. DELIBERATE PROVOCATIVE EXPOSURE TESTING

After the five days of avoidance, foods are tested as single meals. No restriction is made on quantity of food during these test meals. In a high carbohydrate food, the blood glucose is tested at forty-five minutes. Other foods are tested at one hour. A micromethod is used which requires one or two drops of blood from a finger. Each morning the blood sugar is taken to determine if there is a proper baseline of less than 110 mg percent. If there is a blood sugar of 160 mg percent or beyond during a test meal, then the blood sugar is taken again before the next test meal. Testing is not done until the blood sugar normalizes to 110 mg percent or less. A blood sugar of 160 mg percent or beyond at any time postmeal is considered abnormal.

If the person has hypertension or hypotension, the blood pressure is taken before each meal and one hour after each meal. The pulse is taken before each meal and at fifteen minute intervals up to one hour and a half after each meal. A normal pulse may range from 60 in a well exercised patient to 85 in the majority of patients. An increase or decrease in pulse from the original baseline is considered significant.

It is best to take the temperature using a biofeedback thermometer. The temperature is taken in the fingers of the left hand before the meal is eaten and periodically after the meal, especially at one hour. If the temperature drops, it suggests a reaction. If the food is metabolically handled properly, the temperature usually increases a few degrees. The patient eats four meals a day—three in the office and one at home. A serum insulin spot check is made on certain foods when the blood sugar is high. Three hours later a urine sample is given and tested for vitamin C. This will often reveal that vitamin C is deficient after such a reaction. A spot check is also made on blood insulin after a person has reacted to a food with hyperglycemia. If the patient is an insulin dependent diabetic, test the first food in the morning before insulin is given. If a hyperglycemic reaction to the test food does not occur, or normalization of blood sugar after the test does occur within a couple of hours, then insulin is not administered. Testing should continue. In some insulin dependent patients, it becomes mandatory to provide insulin after this first test meal. However, it should be understood that two thirds of those considered to be insulin dependent at the beginning of the examination turn out not to be insulin dependent by means of this examination.

In deliberate provocative food testing, there are several options that need to be considered:

A. Use of market grown foods with the potential of insecticide residues.

B. Use of less chemically contaminated foods (i.e., organic foods).

C. Raw foods.

D. Cooked foods.

E. Sprouted seeds and so forth.

Some ecologists have specialized in basic testing with less chemically contaminated foods. This is the standard of excellence and absolutely necessary in some cases. However, for many the market grown vegetables and meats can be satisfactorily used for testing. Each time a food undergoes change (for example, milk made into a cheese, cooking, sprouting), it needs to be tested as a separate food.

Consideration of Subjective and Objective Testing: It should be understood that hyperglycemia, as a manifestation of maladaptive allergic-like reactions, is a reflection of pancreatic malfunction. The disease process in relationship to a maladaptive reaction to a specific food or chemical always involves pancreatic inhibition. Any organ system, however, can be affected. Therefore, Bio-Ecologic observations should include all organ systems and objective and subjective symptoms. Peripheral temperature, saliva pH, pulse and motor strength provide readily assessable objective observations. Motor strength can be tested by judging the strength of opposing thumb and little finger or an outstretched arm.

Symptoms to look for during testing of foods and chemicals:

Joints: ache/pain, stiffness, swelling, erythema/warmth/redness

Skin: itching local/general, scratching, moist/sweating, flushing/hives, pallor/white or ghostly

Head pain: headache mild/moderate, severe migraine, ache/pressure, tight/explode, throbbing/stabbing

Fatigue: tired, generalized heaviness, sleepy/yawning, exhausted, fall asleep

Generalized: dizzy/lightheaded, imbalance/staggering, going to faint, vertigo/blackout, chilly/cold, warmth/hot flashes

Depressed: withdrawn/listless, vacant/dull faces, negative/indifferent, confused/dazed, depressed, crying/sobbing

Stimulated: silly/intoxicated, grimacing, more alert/talkative, hyperactive, tense/restless, anxious/apprehensive, fear/panic, irritable/angry

Speech comprehension: mentally sluggish, concentration poor, memory loss (acute), speech slurred, stammering/stuttering, speech paralysis/loss of, reads aloud poorly, reads without comprehension, hears without comprehension, math/spelling errors

Muscle: muscle tremor/jerking, muscle cramps/spasms, pseudoparalysis/weak

Contact: poor contact, surroundings unreal, disoriented/catatonic/stuporous, false belief/delusion/hallucination/to wander in mind/false perception, suicidal/feel like hurting self, maniacal/very highly disturbed

Muscles: tight/stiff, ache/sore/pain, neck/trapezius, upper/lower back, upper/lower extremities

Nasal: sneezed/urge to, itching/rubbing, obstruction, discharge, postnasal drip, sinus discomfort, stuffy feeling

Throat, mouth: itching, sore/tight/swollen, dysphagia/difficulty in swallowing/choking, weak voice/hoarse, salivation/mucus, bad/metallic taste

Ears: itching, full/blocked, drythema of pinna (reddening), tinnitis/ringing in ears, earache, hearing loss, hyperacusis/abnormal sensitivity to sound

Lungs, heart: coughing, wheezing, reduced air flow, retracting/sob, heavy/tight, not enough air, hyperventilation/rapid breathing, chest pain, tachycardia/rapid pulse, palpitations/rapid, violent or throbbing pulse

Vision: blurring, acuity decreased, spots/flashes, darker/vision loss, photophobia/brighter, diplopia/double vision, dyslexia/difficulty reading/transposition of similar letters/letters or words becoming small or large, words moving around

Eyes: itch/burn/pain, lacrimation/tearing, injected/FB sensitivity, allergic shiners, feel heavy

G-U: voided/mild urge, frequency, urgency/pressure, painful or difficult urination, dysuria/genital itch

G-I-Abdomen: nausea, belching, full/bloated, vomiting, pressure/pain/cramps, flatus/rumbling, BM/diarrhea, gall bladder symptoms, hunger/thirst, hyperacidity

5. INTRADERMAL AND/OR SUBLINGUAL SERIAL DILUTION TESTING OF SPECIFIC ITEMS

This kind of testing usually constitutes twenty to thirty items such as molds, cat, dog, grasses, trees and so forth. From these tests, neutralization doses are made. A few patients who are highly reactive to foods are provided neutralization doses. This improves their state of addiction and their ability to be on a rotation diet.

6. INHALATION TESTING

Petrochemical hydrocarbons and ammonia are sniffed for a five minute period, the pulse and blood pressure having been recorded before beginning the test and again upon the finish of the test. The mental and physical state is also monitored closely.

7. CYTOTOXIC TESTING

The cytotoxic study is a subjective study of the relative fragility and sensitivity of blood cells, particularly white blood cells, to food and chemical antigens or extracts.

8. TOTAL IgE AND RAST

The total IgE is run before the RAST test. If it is low, about twelve items are run as a routine including common grasses, trees, foods, household mites and so forth.

If the total IgE is high, then a large assortment of tests are done on the RAST. From this testing, an optimum dose schedule of hyposensitization is arranged.

Within the first two days, a cytotoxic blood test for foods and chemicals is run. This consists of microscopic evidence of injury to cells on exposure to food particles. A cytotoxic test is not considered to be an allergy test but is instead a medical test revealing specifically the response of

blood cells to foods or chemicals. It is a reflection of the
current state of the homeostatic metabolic balance and
reveals maladaptivity that might otherwise be missed with
other types of examinations. It does not necessarily parallel
evidences of maladaptivity discovered in other organ
systems.

9. PHENOLIC FOOD COMPOUND TESTING

This test consists of provoking symptoms by administering
differing concentrations of phenolic food compounds, such
as gallic acid, cinnamic acid, anthocyanidins, phenyl
isothiocyanate, phloridzin, naphthoquinones, coumarins,
apicol/eucenol, indole, and flavonols. When symptoms appear
testing is continued until a neutralizing dose is determined.

Treatment consists of gradually increasing doses of
phenolic food compounds for tolerance staying below the
reactive state. This test likely functions on the principle of
evoking enzyme production. Another possibility is that of
an immunologic reaction evoking haptens formation and
that the graduated doses act as a desensitization of the
immunologic reaction. We have been encouraged by the
relief patients have received by this process.

Candida Albicans infection assessment: Blood is drawn
for a serum Candida precipitin test. Samples from
the nose, throat, arm pits, genital area, vagina, rectal area
and from inside the rectum are taken for culturing. Also,
Candida albicans is always intradermal tested, and if positive, neutralization doses are arranged.

Bacterial cultures for autogenous vaccines: A routine
culture from the nose and throat may be made; the
bacteria that is grown is combined for an autogenous
vaccine. If the patient has infections anywhere else, such
as on the skin or in the urinary tract, a specific autogenous
vaccine is made from these areas.

Instruments used in bio-ecologic testing:

A. The Model YSI23A Glucose Analyzer is the only glucose micromethod not influenced by the amount of Vitamin C in the blood. It is suitable for clinic or hospital. It is manufactured by Yellow Springs Instrument Company, Yellow Springs, Ohio 45387.

B. StatTek instrument by Bio-Dynamics with StatTek test strips and Autolet.

C. Ames Dextrometer—a sensitive electronic instrument using Dextrostrips and microlances.

D. Ames Glucometer—a valuable instrument for home use. Diabetics should have a home instrument.

E. Autolet with Monolet lancets by Monoject, a division of Sherwood Medical, for home use. Test for glucose using the Chemstrip bG for whole blood by Bio-Dynamics. The finger is pricked with Microlance, a blood lancet by Becton-Dickinson Co.

F. Temperature—biofeedback thermometer by Curtin Matheson Scientific, Inc. Waterbath thermometer by Curtin Matheson Scientific, Inc., P.O. Box 1546, Houston, Texas, 77001. Thermometer ring by Futurehealth, Inc., Dept. P-100, P.O. Box 947, Bensalem, PA 19020.

G. pH paper—Insta-Check Hydrion pH by Micro Lab, Inc. Use double cartridge with 6–8 on one side and 5.2–6.6 on the other side.

H. Stethoscope and sphygmomanometer—we use a stethoscope to count heartbeat for one minute.

The following basic information is in the process of being integrated into clinical practice:

A. The role of lipid metabolism and prostaglandins.

B. The role of phenolic food compounds. Where possible, it is wise to isolate reactions to specific classes of substances found in multiple foods such as a generalized reaction to gluten found in several cereal grains or reactions to phenol ring substances found in many foods and chemical contaminants. Phenol rings comprise several amino acids (aromatic amino acids including phenylalanine, tyrosine and tryptophan) and their products. Petrochemical compounds frequently contain phenol ring compounds. Phenol is a common preservative used in medication. It is also used to kill microorganisms for vaccines and found in artificial colors and so forth. Provocative testing to chemical contaminants containing phenol and plant phenolic substances reveals frequent sensitivities. These reactions evoke an assortment of physical and central nervous system maladaptive responses. Decarboxylation products of phenolic foods contain an assortment of biologically active compounds capable of disordering metabolic functions. A classic example is the high level of tyromine found in cheddar cheese and responsible for headaches in those hypersensitive to tyromine.[1] Several have raised the question of significance of these phenolic compounds in evoking nonimmunologic metabolic disorders as well as immunologic reactions through hapten formation.[2]

Our observations are that chronic heavy exposure to phenol and similar phenolic compounds, whether in foods or chemical contaminants, can exceed the metabolic capacity of tolerance of an individual and thus lead to inhibition of the enzymes which process these compounds. It is our postulation that addiction is also a state that disorders the necessary enzyme function needed to process these compounds. So far, we are impressed that by the time the disease process has advanced to the clinical diabetes mellitus stage, there exists a universal enzyme inhibition producing a hypersensitivity to phenolics. The rule is that with the establishment of a nonaddicted, appropriately nourished and optimum exercised state, these hypersensitive reactions to phenolics disappear or are materially reduced. Supplemental cysteine has been observed to reduce phenolic caused symptoms in related cases. However, it is possible that some will not spontaneously recover their enzymatic function necessary for handling these compounds, and therefore, need the benefit of hyposensitization treatment. The most likely cause of hypersensitive response stems from the enzyme fatiguing effect of chronic heavy exposure. This is capable of occurring if optimum conditions for enzyme function are also present such as the necessary nutrient cofactors, optimum pH and temperature, and so on. This is best achieved by providing a small dose of varied plant phenolic substances starting with a nonreactive dose (neutralization dose) and gradually increasing the dose over weeks or months until a one milligram dose can be tolerated. Hyposensitization can rapidly occur by three sublingual exposures a day. R. W. Gardner and his associates have been making a detailed study of these possibilities.[3]

C. The role of dehydroascorbic acid. Dehydroascorbic acid and dehydroascorbic are in equilibrium. Most authors refer to this collectively as dehydroascorbic acid. At the cell membrane level, dehydroascorbic serves the purpose of transport through the cell membrane and is reduced to ascorbic acid within the cell.[4] We are concerned with disordered metabolic states that interfere with this normal function of dehydroascorbic. The result is a rise in serum dehydroascorbic toxicity. Researchers suggest that elevated dehydroascorbic acid exerts a number of toxic effects including autonomic dysfunction, slowed cell division, lymphocytolysis and thymic involution, lipid peroxidation, complexing with SH groups and ascorbic acid-dehydroascorbic redox potential shift in the oxidative direction.[5]

In infectious diseases, blood ascorbic acid decreases and dehydroascorbic acid increases.[6] Pharmacological doses of dehydroascorbic acid are reported to be diabetogenic.[7] Animal experiments indicate large doses of dehydroascorbic acid degenerate the beta cells of the pancreas.[8] Serum dehydroascorbic acid is reported to be continuously elevated in patients with diabetes mellitus.[9] Fetal malformations in diabetes[10] likely result from hyperglycemia interfering with ascorbic acid-dehydroascorbic acid cellular homeostasis.[11] A likely formulation is that addiction and associated infections disorder the metabolic handling of ascorbic acid and dehydroascorbic acid. This leads to a disordered state of metabolism in which ascorbic acid is oxidized to dehydroascorbic acid; this then adversely affects pancreatic beta cells and many other possible body and central nervous system functions.

Bio-ecologic treatment

The principal Bio-Ecologic method is to treat broadly and simultaneously as many factors as possible that have both major and minor relationships to the disease state. Usually, treatment does not occur during the testing period. Exceptions to this rule are: insulin dependence, rare management needs for tranquilizers, antiseizure medication, antiasthma medication, cardiac medication and so forth. Where indicated, we give behavioral training, Sedac or myoflex treatments (forms of electrostimulation) for tension and insomnia, and sometimes electric shock treatment for a persistent deep depression or psychosis. There are frequent interviews and twice weekly group sessions for meeting educational and motivational needs. The testing program requires four weeks. During the fourth week, the laboratory work is assessed, nutrients are arranged and a diversified rotation diet specific to the patient's test evidence is planned.

DIVERSIFIED ROTATION
DIET AND PROTEIN, FAT,
CARBOHYDRATE RATIOS

A discussion of the diversified rotation diet is presented in chapter four. This diet is the most central of all therapies; for the diversified rotation diet prevents food addiction from existing. This diet reverses and prevents the progression of the basic addictive stress-evoked disease process.

Our observations are that diabetes disorders protein metabolism, and therefore contrary to popular medical opinion and practice, the diabetic does better on a low protein diet of 10 to 20 percent of total calories rather than a high protein diet. Specific demonstrated amino acid deficiencies should be supplemented. The most appropriate diet appears most likely to be on the order of 10 to 20 percent protein, 10 to 20 percent fat (i.e., the largely saturated and transfats commonly used) with the rest complex carbohydrates. Free (simple) sugars should be reserved for occasional treats only. What appears as an exception to this is the usually useful addition of one teaspoon of nonheated honey (organic) premeal on each fourth day. Nonheated honey is a valuable source of proteases which in turn exert control over prostaglandins and by this mechanism aid in preventing hyperglycemia. The lipids used by most people contain saturated fats and translinoleic acid, both of which are detrimental if taken in amounts beyond 10 to 20 percent. However, cis-linoleic acid and gamma-linolenic acid are useful in reversing arteriosclerosis and therefore are not considered in this low fat percentage. Cis-linoleic acid and gamma-linolenic acid can be used as supplements beyond the 10 to 20 percent fat in the diet. These cold pressed oils should be kept refrigerated once opened. Vitamin E is best taken as 400 IU three times a day to prevent peroxidation of these unsaturated lipids. At least the above proportions of protein, fats and complex carbohydrates has proved useful in Western culture. We still have to consider other cultures such as the Greenland Eskimos doing well on a raw fish diet which is high in both cis-linoleic acid and protein and low in carbohydrates (simple and complex). It is likely that the high cis-linoleic acid is the great protector in this diet. Since Western culture diets are not high in fish, the food tolerance is arranged otherwise.

NUTRITIONAL SUPPLEMENT CONSIDERATIONS

The paramecium study of twelve vitamins is studied. If a vitamin is significantly low, it is given three times a day. If it is normal, it is given usually once a day for an initial two to three months. If B12 is low, it is given intramuscularly or sublingually as 1000 mcg once or twice a week. This is usually associated with 10 mg of folic acid. If beta-carotene is high, it usually represents tyrosine deficiency. Vitamin C is given as 4 grams three times a day. Vitamin C is best taken on arising and between meals so as not to interfere with mineral absorption since purposely more is being given than absorbed and some minerals would be retained in the nonabsorbed vitamin C. If the hair test reveals low sodium, it can then be administered as sodium ascorbate. If there is high sodium, it should be administered as ascorbic acid. If given as ascorbic acid, it can be given half an hour ahead of the meal or with the meal. If given as sodium ascorbate, it can be given thirty minutes after the meal. It is better not to give this with the meal, since sodium ascorbate is an alkalinizing agent. Sometimes, ascorbates for potassium, magnesium and calcium are administered. If these are used as a mineral source, they should be given thirty minutes after the meal, since they are alkalinizing. The alkalinizing capacity will aid the digestive process of providing the optimum pH for pancreatic enzyme function.

B6 is given as either pyridoxine, 500 mg, or even better, as pyridoxal-5-phosphate, 50 mg. If either kynurenic acid or xanthurenic acid is high, B6 is given three times a day. In the majority of cases B6 is needed at a rate of three times a day. In the rare situation where there is no specific evidence of need, it is administered once a day. Most of the time, the paramecium study reveals a normal B6; a high kynurenic acid and xanthurenic acid will be present approximately 80 percent of the time. Since B6 is a cofactor in so many enzyme reactions, the amino acid profile provides several internal evidences of a B6 deficiency and/or utilization disorder. B6 can best be administered sublingually by emptying the powder from the capsule under the tongue.

B2 is administered in approximately equal doses with B6. It should be given as a phosphorylated B2. This form is better tolerated than the nonphosphorylated B2. It is given as 50 mg three times a day. Seldom do any paramecium studies reveal B2 deficiency.

B1 is occasionally deficient on the paramecium study or transketolase study. It usually is given as powder in a capsule of 100 mg three times a day and can be sublingually absorbed during the meal.

B3 is administered either as niacinamide or niacin, usually as 500 mg. It is commonly demonstrated as deficient or low normal on a paramecium study. It is well to give B3 as 500 mg three times a day irrespective of what the paramecium study states, simply because it is a methyl absorber. It is imperative to give it when administering tyrosine.

B5 is administered as pantothenic acid. It is seldom deficient on the paramecium study. It is usually administered as 500 mg once a day.

Para-amino benzoic acid is not on the paramecium study. It is usually given as 500 mg three times a week. It is especially useful in reducing the aging process.

B12 can be administered orally as 1000 mcg three times a day. If it is well within normal range, it is given as once a day. If low normal, it is administered three times a day. If specifically abnormal, it is administered as an injection or as a sublingual use of the injectable solution on a once to twice a week basis. This dose is in addition to the 1000 mcg three times a week taken as the powder.

Folic acid on the paramecium study is deficient between 50 to 60 percent of the time. This parallels quite well the spillage of formiminoglutamic acid in the urine (FIGLU test) during the stress day. Folic acid is usually administered as a powder slightly below one mg. At one mg and more, folic acid is a prescription item. If deficient, this is given three times a day and may range from one to five capsules, depending on the need. It is best absorbed sublingually by emptying the powder under the tongue during a meal.

The sublingual administration of B-complex vitamins markedly improves the absorption of the vitamin. Usually, the meal sufficiently masks the taste of the vitamin so as not to interfere with this method. If need be, a drop of honey can be placed on the tongue to mask the taste of the vitamins. For most people honey can be used frequently. Honey that has not been heated (heating destroys proteases) can be used, and different honeys can be selected for each day so that they can be rotated. The use of honey is often demonstrated to be possible for diabetics.

Minerals are judged from serum studies of calcium, magnesium, potassium, copper, zinc, manganese and sometimes chromium as well as a hair test biopsy of calcium, magnesium, copper, potassium, chromium, manganese and selenium.

Calcium, if deficient in the blood, strongly suggests the need for supplementation. It also may represent a parathyroid deficiency. A seldom seen deficiency of calcium in the hair indicates a nutritional intake deficiency. More often, there is an excess of calcium in the hair. This does not mean that there really is an excess of calcium in the blood; it merely means that there is an excess deposit of calcium in the hair. This condition almost routinely exists in hypoparathyroidism: there is low calcium in the blood but high calcium being deposited both in the hair and in the bones. If there is no internal evidence of calcium deficiency and there is high calcium in the hair, this would be an indication that calcium need not be supplemented. When supplementing calcium, doses range from 500 mg once a day to three times a day. Considerably higher doses of calcium, plus the administration of one of the synthetic vitamin Ds (ergocalciferol or dihydrotachysterol) should be given in hypoparathyroidism.

Magnesium is judged by both serum and hair. If both are low, it is positive evidence of nutritional need. If the magnesium is normal in the blood and high in the hair, it is indicative of no particular need for magnesium supplementation. However, another way of judging magnesium levels is by seeing whether there are any enzymes in the amino acid profile that use magnesium. Magnesium should be supplemented irrespective of normal evidence as judged by serum studies or by the hair study. Usual dosage ranges from 90 mg once to three times a day.

Potassium is judged by both blood and hair, and if either shows a deficiency, it should be supplemented. The usual supplement dose is 90 mg three times a day. This may be administered as potassium ascorbate, as potassium bicarbonate or as a chelated potassium.

Copper is judged by both blood and hair analysis, and if either is deficient, it should be supplemented. It is usually supplemented as 2 to 5 mg three times a day as a chelate.

Zinc is judged by an assay of blood and hair, and if either is deficient, it should be supplemented. As a chelate, it could be administered as 10 to 30 mg a day or as a 10 percent zinc sulfate, 75 mg a day, given in divided doses as drops under the tongue (five drops, three times a day).

Manganese is judged by both blood and hair, and if either is deficient, it should be supplemented. It is frequently deficient in the hair, even though it is normal in the blood. Where manganese is used, there are also frequent internal evidences on the amino acid profile revealing weak enzyme functions. Therefore, there is reason to believe that manganese is a frequently deficient mineral. This can be administered as a chelate, 10 to 30 mg a day. It can be administered as a 1 to 10 percent solution of manganese chloride, 7.5 to 75 mg a day as indicated. It can be administered in divided doses as drops for sublingual absorption (five drops, three times a day). The most appropriate manganese is a manganese-arginine chelate.

Selenium is tested in the hair, and if deficient or low normal, should be administered. It can be administered as a yeast source or as a kelp source. Most people will tolerate the kelp better. The usual dose is 50 to 150 mg a day.

Lithium is tested in the hair. If low, a supplement can be given of lithium carbonate, 250 mg a day. It is seldom needed.

The best method of mineral absorption is sublingual. Sublingual formulas can be used as powders administered during the meal in the same way that the B-complex vitamins are administered. Ascorbates of calcium, potassium and magnesium are available and are good sources for mineral administration.

Iron is tested in both the serum and hair. If there is a deficiency in either, iron should be administered orally. If iron is deficient in the serum, it should be administered as a liver-iron combination intramuscularly on a once a week basis. This should be combined with the oral administration. Iron can be administered as a chelate of 10 mg three times a day or as an iron sulfate in a delayed action capsule at 150 mg once a day. It is best to give the iron at the time that vitamin C is being administered. Vitamin C enhances absorption, so care is advised to prevent toxicity.

The heavy metals, mercury, lead, arsenic and cadmium, are tested in the hair. If these are high, it has been observed that 12 grams of vitamin C supplemented a day will chelate out these minerals. If lead or mercury is exceptionally high, it might be wise to do an EDTA chelation and discover the amount spilled in the urine in twenty-four hours. Occasionally, EDTA chelation is indicated for these heavy metals.

If and when phosphorylated compounds such as Pyridoxal-5 Phosphate, phosphorylated B2, phosphorylated B1 or phosphorus-containing substances such as lecithin are used they should be separated from the mineral supplements. It is suggested that mineral supplements be taken at breakfast and bedtime while phosphorus substances be taken at noon and evening meals.

AMINO ACID SUPPLEMENTATION

The need for amino acid supplementation is determined by the amino acid profile. The optimum use of this profile can best be given by a chemist assessing the enzyme systems in the amino acid profile. From this, recommendations can be made for specific amino acid supplements as well as the internal evidence of the need for specific cofactors (vitamins, minerals, amino acids) and citric acid. It is common to find a citric acid cycle disorder, which is thought to be more often than not a manifestation of low alpha-ketoglutaric acid. This is judged by evidence of low glutamic acid, since alpha-ketoglutaric acid is one of its precursors. Also, high alpha-aminoadipic acid would give evidence of low alpha-ketoglutaric acid, since both B6 and alpha-ketoglutaric acid are needed in the change of alpha-aminoadiptic acid to alpha-ketoadiptic acid.

Disordered urea cycle metabolism is quite frequent, and the most frequent disorder is high ornithine. This would be indicative of an enzymatic weakness of turning ornithine into citrulline and/or also ornithine into glutamic acid. The lysinemic pathway frequently shows evidence of disorder. There are at least nine possibilities involving the uric acid cycle and lysine pathways which can demonstrate the need for reducing proteins to 10 to 20 percent of the total calories included in any single meal.

There is internal evidence that bouts of hyperammonemia are quite frequent in this disordered ability to handle a high protein intake. The inability to turn ammonia into urea with normal facilitation occurs also in response to a state of acidosis. This acid state is characteristic of the withdrawal phase of addiction. Vitamin C becomes an important issue in these cases, because it can tie up ammonia. Such is the fact whether the high ammonia is caused by a disordered liver function, a disordered balance between glutamic acid and glutamine or a production of ammonia by bacterial action in the colon. Adequate vitamin C should also be available as a detoxifying agent.

Frequently, one sees a disordered methionine metabolism. Homocystinuria, which would be characteristic of folic acid, B12 and B6 deficiency, also is closely related to a methionine metabolism disorder. Cystathioninuria is not uncommon.

The disordered methionine metabolism produces methylated amines. These methylated amines produce toxins but also by demand create deficiencies in the branch-chained amino acids and B3.

Frequently, supplementations are needed for the following: glutamic acid, valine, leucine, isoleucine, phenylalanine, tyrosine, cystine and citric acid. Many of the amino acids can be obtained as single amino acids or in appropriate groups. Amino acids are usually administered as 1 to 3 grams. Citric acid can be administered in 5 to 8 grams in five divided doses. Sometimes, it is more appropriately administered as a combined citric acid-aspartic acid. This last combination is the preferred method of administering citric acid, unless aspartic acid is higher than normal.

Tryptophan can be useful when associated with adequate B6, to reduce myoclonus or insomnia and may be administered in 3 to 6 gram doses at bedtime.

Tyrosine is a precursor to the thyroid hormone; it appears that it is more often needed than thyroid when the following symptoms are present: weakness, low temperature and low blood pressure. Three to 6 grams a day in divided doses may correct this syndrome. If not, then thyroid should be used. High beta-carotene suggests that there is either a tyrosine deficiency or a thyroid deficiency. Thyroid hormone is necessary for the liver to turn beta-carotene into vitamin A. An excess of beta-carotene is the most frequent finding. Tyrosine is also useful as an antidepressant. It is also a precursor to dopamine, and therefore is useful for the restless leg syndrome. For this syndrome, it is usually administered as 500 to 1500 mg at bedtime. Since supplementing tyrosine makes a greater demand for B3, it is wise to simultaneously give niacinamide, 500 to 1500 mg per day.

It is wise for a biochemist to provide a reading on the amino acid studies along with the associated lab work. One organization devoted to such a service is Bionostics, P.O. Drawer 400, Lisle, IL 60532.

VACCINATIONS

Reduced resistance to microorganisms is characteristic of the diabetes mellitus disease process. For a reinstatement of normal immunological defense against opportunist microorganisms, it is best to grow bacteria from the nose, throat, skin lesions and infected urine and then make autogenous vaccines. These are administered by gradually increasing the dose and giving it subcutaneously once a week and then three days later giving the same dose sublingually. Useful stock vaccines

routinely used are Rhus-All and BCG. In selective
cases, the addition of influenza and pneumococcus is
also used.

MICROORGANISM MANAGEMENT

Acute bacterial infections of sinuses, ears, skin, urine and so
forth often need an internal course of appropriate antibiotics. An antibiotic bacterial sensitivity study identifies the
appropriate antibiotics.

Fungus infections should be vigorously treated. Candida
albicans when cultured should be treated with Nystatin
oral solution, oral tablets and vaginal tablets or powder. The
initial treatment requires a minimum of one month. Occasionally, there are cases in which immunocompetence against
Candida albicans cannot be restored. In these cases, Nystatin
is required on a maintenance basis. Vaccine therapy as
optimum dose therapy (neutralization) should be used whenever intradermal testing reveals a reaction. It should not be
considered adequate to handle a Candida albicans infection
without an initial antibiotic treatment. Several researchers
have found homeopathic doses of Candida albicans to be more
satisfactory than the serial dilution neutralization dose.

Nizarol (Ketoconazole) is necessary for some in the
treatment of candida albicans. This is given as a 200 mg
tablet daily for several months.

EXERCISE

Daily exercise is needed to stimulate numerous metabolic
functions and to oxygenate tissues. This is best provided by
lightly jogging (loping) or brisk walking one-half hour in
the morning before breakfast. Equivalents are bicycling,
tennis and similar sports.

TREATMENT PRIORITIES

The last thing to give a diabetic is insulin. The first thing
to do for a diabetic is to reverse the disease process. This is

accomplished by understanding its dynamics (i.e., reversal of addiction, optimum nutrition and supplemental proteases and bicarbonate). Insulin is provided only when optimum correction of the disordered metabolism does not demonstrate sufficient reversal of the disease process. It is also given to those people who refuse to follow the prescribed physiological corrective lifestyle.

REFERENCES

1. Newberne, P. M. 1980. Naturally occurring food-borne toxicants. In *Modern Nutrition in Health and Disease*. R. S. Goodhart and M. E. Shils, eds. Philadelphia: Lea and Febiger, pp. 463–96.

2. Agharanya, J. C., Alonso, R. and Wurtman, R. J. 1981. Changes in catecholamine excretion after short-term tyrosine ingestion in normally fed human subjects. *American Journal of Clinical Nutrition* 34:82; Berger, P. S. 1981. Biochemistry and the schizophrenias —old concepts and new hypotheses. *Journal of Nervous and Mental Disease* 169:90; Fairbairn, J. W., ed. 1959. *The Pharmacology of Plant Phenolics*. New York: Academic Press; Freedman, S. O., et al. 1962. Identification of a simple chemical compound (chlorogenic acid) as an allergen in plant materials causing human atopic disease. *American Journal of Medical Science* 244:548; Lovenberg, W. 1973. Some vaso- and psychoactive substances in foods; amines, stimulants, depressants and hallucinogens. In *Toxicants Occurring Naturally in Foods*. Washington, DC: National Academy of Science; Ribereau-Gayon, P. 1972. *Plant Phenolics*. New York; Hafner Publishing: Robinson, T. 1980. *The Organic Constituents of Higher Plants, Their Chemistry and Interrelationships*. Cordus Press; Singleton, V. S. and Kratzer, F. H. 1969. Toxicity and related physiological activity of phenolic substances of plant origin. *Journal of Agricultural Food Chemistry* 17:497.

3. Gardner, R. W., McGovern, J. J., Jr. and Brenneman, L. D. April 4–8, 1981. The role of plant and animal phenyls in food allergy. The American College of Allergists, 37th Annual Congress, Washington, D.C.

4. Lewin, S. 1976. *Vitamin C: Its Molecular Biology and Medical Potential*. New York: Academic Press, figure 1.4.

5. Ely, J. T. A. 1981. Personal communication.

6. Chakrabarti, B. and Banerjee, S. 1955. Dehydroascorbic acid level in blood of patients suffering from various infectious diseases. *Proceedings of the Society for Experimental Biological Medicine* 88:581–83.

7. Patterson, J. W. 1950. *Journal of Biological Chemistry* 183:81–88.

8. MacDonald, M. K. and Bhattacharya, S. K. 1956. *Quarterly Journal of Experimental Physiology* 41(2):153–61.

9. Chatterjee, I. B., Majumber, A. K., Nanadi, B. K., et al. 1975. Synthesis and some major functions of vitamin C in animals. *Annals of the New York Academy of Science* 244:548.

10. Miller, E., Hare, J. W., Cloherty, J. P., et al. 1981. Elevated maternal hemoglobin A1C in early pregnancy and major congenital anomalies in infants of diabetic mothers. *New England Journal of Medicine* 304:1331–34.

11. Mann, G. V. 1974. Hypothesis: the role of vitamin C in diabetic angiopathy. *Perspectives of Biological Medicine* 4:210–17; Mann, G. V. and Newton, P. 1975. The membrane transport of ascorbic acid. *Annals of the New York Academy of Science* 258:243–52; Ely, J. T. A. Oct. 1, 1981. Hyperglycemia and major congenital anomalies. *New England Journal of Medicine.*

Anatomy of resistance to the emergent paradigm: orthomolecular medicine

Resistance to Bio-Ecologic treatment modalities persists in the 1980s throughout the medical community. Helen First, Ph.D., in a cogent and illuminating article, published in the **Journal of Orthomolecular Psychiatry,** *volume 9, number 4, 1980, presents some valid reasons for the existence of this phenomenon, and indicates signposts toward a more hopeful future. Dr. First is Clinical Associate Professor of Psychiatry and Human Behavior (Retired) at Jefferson Medical College, Thomas Jefferson University.*

The Problem: Cultural indicators of a growing concern with nutrition and resistance to that concern

Public views of doctors include, self-evidently, the way doctors themselves view their colleagues, specifically their colleagues who practice orthomolecular medicine or orthomo-

lecular psychiatry. Resistance to the orthomolecular concept, that form of health care whose core principle is the
maintenance of health by means of "providing the cells
with the right molecules in optimum amounts" (Pauling,
1968), persists even though cultural indicators confirm that
the climate of opinion is changing. Everywhere there is an
exploding new interest in diet. The Director of The
National Cancer Institute agrees that "on the basis of
currently available evidence the adoption of nutritional
guidelines is warranted" (N.Y. Times). The President and
Director of The Sloan-Kettering Institute acknowledges the
relationship of nutrition to immunity and cancer in a review
of the subject (Good, 1979). A U.S. Senate Investigating
Committee report is published on Diet Related to Killer
Diseases (U.S. Govt., 1977). The New England Journal of
Medicine maintains an ongoing concern with nutrition. The
Sciences, Journal of The New York Academy of Sciences,
sums up an article, "Food for Thought," with "Findings
show that diet does indeed play a direct role in brain
function."

In the light of this expanding awareness of the nutrition-
brain/mind axis, the persistence of the medical establishment's resistance to the orthomolecular concept calls for a
comprehensive examination and explication, which is precisely what this paper aims to do. First, I will indicate the
dynamics of resistance with examples from present and past
history of medicine. Second, I will demonstrate how
medical paradigms are evolved out of the repetitive struggle
between tradition and innovation, with the tension between them being a measure of the resistance which only
time can resolve. Third, I will show how the present
resistance is informed by the specific etiology paradigm,
now becoming obsolescent, and, finally, looking to the
future, I shall suggest what the orthomolecular paradigm has
to offer for research and for true preventive medicine.

The term orthomolecular is defined as "designating the
normal constituents of the body including substances
formed endogenously and those acquired through diet." The
"normal constituents of the body" used therapeutically

include vitamins, metals and trace minerals, amino acids, and enzymes. In addition, every effort is made to rid the body of toxins, allergens, contaminants from within or without and to prevent recontamination.

In its resistance to this commonsense approach to health care the medical establishment has shown every reaction from mild disinterest to the vindictive and irresponsible deception of the authors of the APA Task Force on Vitamin Therapy in Psychiatry (Megavitamin, 1973). To comprehend such deportment on the part of people who as scientists are expected to act in a manner that is honorable, unbiased, and above all intelligent, it is useful to review what communication research indicates are some of the problems involved in introducing new ideas and changing public opinion (Fishbein, 1967; McGuire, 1967; Pool, 1973; Rhine, 1967). Then we can begin to identify by their performances how and why objectors to the orthomolecular concept act out their predictable scripts.

Dynamics of influence according to communication theory and resistances to the process

The first requisite for an exchange of opinion according to communication theory is an audience, but many of the channels by which a message can be conveyed are studiously and cunningly blocked by the opposition. One out of countless examples of this maneuver is the attempt to delimit the audience for the *Journal of Orthomolecular Psychiatry* by having it omitted from the *Index Medicus*. This restraint on the dissemination of scientific information was engineered by a government bureaucrat who also served on the APA Task Force. The Journal flourishes, nonetheless, with the creditable record of having a hundred library subscribers, and a reader circulation that compares favorably with the top psychiatric journals. Also, it is included in *Current Content*, another service index for

medical literature. The transparent reason given for exclud-
ing the Journal was that the Index, which abstracts about
2300 journals, was not geared to include one more.

Another determining factor in effective influence is the
attractiveness of the source of the message but efforts to
discredit the source have ranged from mindless devaluations
to outright libel. Even the charismatic Linus Pauling is not
immune to such efforts to denigrate the source. Physicians
and others who have never been exposed in person to Dr.
Pauling's incisive thinking and lucid extempore dialectics
have been known, with an air of conspiratorial mockery,
to make snide inferences about his mental status on the
basis of his age, thus denigrating orthomolecular medicine
by dishonoring the originator of the term itself.

Besides an open channel and the acknowledged exper-
tise of the communicator, other factors which determine the
effectiveness of a communication involve the receiver of
the message. For the receiver to accept the message he must
feel his self-esteem to be enhanced by it. But a new idea
like orthomolecular nutritional medicine is a criticism and
an embarrassment to the average physician who had no
training in nutrition in medical school. And for the psychiatrist the idea is especially difficult because of his commitment
to the psychogenic etiology of mental disorders. Also, the
psychotherapy he offers provides him with compelling,
interesting work for which he has in-depth training and in
which he has a great investment. Then, too, doctors whose
income would be threatened if patients turned elsewhere for
a different treatment modality are not likely to feel their
self-esteem enhanced by the orthomolecular approach. The
receiver to accept a message must also find that it provides
some significant compensation, like money, a tangible but
apparently insufficiently compelling reward. As one internist expressed his disinterest in orthomolecular practice: "I
don't have time to learn anything new or out of my field
and besides I know enough to make a living. Period."

Acceptance of the message is influenced also by the
discrepancy between the message and what the receiver
believes. The policy of orthomolecular healing, to support

the body's constructive mechanisms, runs counter to current medical practice with its emphasis on suppressing the body's defenses, that is, the symptoms which too often are labeled as the disease. Discomfort in the presence of such discrepancy leads to avoidance by means of dismissing the disturbing influence with put downs like "anecdotal," "unscientific," "no double-blind studies." Avoidance can also be partial, in the form of selective perception. This selective perception was especially apparent in the APA Task Force report as documented by Hoffer and Osmond (1976) who pointed out that the committee reviewed only niacin-B3 studies but not those studies which reflected the full range of treatment modalities. Also in their review of the studies which it did cover, the Task Force *selected* findings so as to be able to claim results that were misleading and false. While asserting that they had "carefully examined the literature produced by megavitamin proponents," they selectively avoided reviewing the major research and literature, particularly the significant textbook, *Orthomolecular Psychiatry* (Hawkins and Pauling, 1973).

The final hurdle to open communication to be noted here, is what is called immunization. If one holds a critical or disrespectful view of a concept on the basis of little knowledge, he is less likely to be persuaded favorably even when the knowledge base is broadened; or if one makes a public statement or commitment against a viewpoint, he is less likely to be converted to the viewpoint he publicly disavowed. M. A. Lipton, Chairman of The Task Force Report Committee, who by his selection of committee members violated all the rules of fair inquiry set forth by the National Academy of Sciences in regard to the avoidance of bias in the formation of committees, had, long before such time as the committee was formed, presented a paper in Los Angeles, California, in which he opposed orthomolecular psychiatry unambiguously, an act which made him immune to opinion change. An editor of a collection of papers on child abuse justified his rejection of a paper dealing with the orthomolecular approach to this problem by protesting: "How could I explain its inclusion to my colleagues when I have made public statements (as a government agent) against orthomolecular psychiatry?" The blinders of immunization allow the wearer to employ any ruse to maintain tunnel vision. A typical ruse employed by avoidant editors is to hide behind the convention of peer review done by unnamed readers whose self-immunizing bias goes unchallenged, a practice readily recognized for the Kafka-esque pretense that it is (Chalmers, 1977; Cole, 1977).

There is yet one other form of immunity to new ideas, immunity which stems from attachment or anchoring to admired figures, teachers, department heads, colleagues. This is referred to in some quarters as the "Old Boy Syndrome." Fear of being thrown out of "the Club" rigidifies "right" thinking and vaccinates against deviance. "The Old Boy" syndrome is exemplified by the aforementioned child abuse editor who is based at Yale University, "A hotbed of antagonism to the orthomolecular position" according to a Gesell Institute informant. Clubbiness can supercede scientific neutrality. Orthomolecular proponents have borne the brunt of countless ostrich maneuvers knowing full well they were blatant deceits. An allergist with impeccable credentials approached local affiliates of national organizations for crippling diseases with an offer to research a problem that would benefit victims of these diseases, at no expense, discomfort or inconvenience to them. From one organization there was no response. The other informed him that the matter had been submitted to a Review Board. After a decent interval he inquired regarding the "Review Board's" decision and learned, inadvertently, that the "Review Board" was a figment of someone's imagination. None existed (Mandell). Linus Pauling (1979) can claim a record of having had six out of seven grant applications for studies on the use of ascorbic acid with cancer patients turned down. At least one grant application was on the basis that the vitamin increased interferon, a finding amply supported by research (Siegel, 1974; Siegel, 1975; Povolotsky, 1979) and that interferon augments the immune response, a widely accepted fact. So why not use vitamin C to increase the cancer patients' interferon-mediated immune response? Too simple. The American Cancer Society is instead spending $2,000,000 to purchase animal interferon from Finland with which it will be able to treat, at the cost of $20,000 per patient, a handful of beneficiaries, when at the cost of about $9.00 a kilo that readily available ascorbic acid could perform the same task for thousands. This maneuver has all the rationality and directness of Tom Sawyer's plan to release himself when tied to his bed not by lifting the corner bedpost but by sawing off its leg and swallowing the sawdust so as to conceal his mode of escape.

Resistances to medical innovation in the past

Modern resistances to innovative ideas have their counterpart throughout medical history. Gregor Mendel's basic principles of heredity were ignored for thirty-five years. Theodore Schwann's finding that yeast was a living organism was forgotten for twenty years because others couldn't replicate his study. Semmelweis's preachment that puerperal fever could be prevented met with hostility and derision, and his reports were commented on in the medical journals only in the columns devoted to medical humor. Pasteur's early discoveries had to wait twenty years for acceptance and he had to resort to showmanship and sensational public demonstrations in order to beat down skepticism and mockery and to win acceptance for his theory of infection and the value of vaccines to combat them. Anesthesia as a means of lessening the pain of childbirth was opposed by the Scottish clergy on the grounds that pain was ordained by The Maker and only when it was argued that God himself placed Adam in a deep slumber for his phenomenal costalectomy did anesthesia for women win acceptance. Florence Nightingale's efforts to establish nursing as a respectable profession for gentlewomen met with resistance. Joseph Goldberger, the

U.S. Public Health Service physician, who in the line of duty risked his life with yellow fever, dengue and typhus, was harassed throughout his pursuit of the cause of pellagra. A year after he established that pellagra was a nutritional deficiency disease, an achievement characterized as "one of the greatest . . . of modern science," a research commission, a prototype for the APA Task Force, reported that there was no connection of any kind between diet and pellagra, that it was an infectious disease traceable to the stable fly. Only through the inordinately courageous gesture by Goldberger and his assistants of injecting into their own bodies the excrement, mucus and scales of the diseased, with no loss of health, was the opposition silenced (Hospital Practice, 1978).

Of time and paradigms

By arranging in perspective these historical examples of resistance to innovative ideas in medicine, one can observe a dimension in attitude change not emphasized by the communication theorists, namely the effect of time, a dimension which operates similarly in other fields, for instance, art. Impressionist paintings, ridiculed at the Paris Exhibition of 1874, today are the world's treasures. Why are ideas so vehemently rejected at the beginning, warmly embraced after twenty-thirty-forty years? The one word answer is prematurity (Stent, 1972). They are ideas that are ahead of their time. When the climate of opinion changes with the passage of time the new idea, no longer discrepant, becomes the very paradigm around which thought is organized anew. Paradigm metamorphosis is the intellectual task of every period (Kuhn, 1970).

In the forward march of civilization each age formulates a world view that enunciates its comprehension of what is reality, of what is man, his essential nature, how it can be expressed, enhanced, modified, healed. On the basis of this world view special interest groups, artists, philosophers, scientists, and physicians in particular create a paradigm, a model that serves them as a framework for their professional directive. As knowledge expands it calls for periodic reorganization of new data into manageable concepts. Each new paradigm is the contraction of that expanding knowledge.

This paradigm or model of reality has great economic value. It centers attention understandably toward consensually understood goals. As an example, again from art history, when Copernicus and Columbus altered man's view of his world from flat to round, artists developed a new awareness of depth perspective so that modeling and chiaroscuro were perfected, replacing flat, two-dimensional representation. Again, when the new dimension of the Freudian unconscious became common coin, Picasso was able to restore primitive flat painting with the bizarre elaborations and distortions which stem from the unconscious.

Now in medicine the paradigms which determine the physicians' driving concern and give explicit direction to the research by which medical knowledge is advanced, these paradigms are informed by new explorations, new advances in biology, physics, chemistry, mathematics, war, industry, technology. It's been a highspeed highway from the stethoscope to computerized axial tomography, and a long one from Moses, the first agent for large scale public health and sanitation, through Hippocrates, the natural healer, to today's climate of magical expectations for specific cures for specific diseases. That rigid concept, that each disease has its specific cause and cure, which Dixon calls the theory of specific etiology, is the paradigm that has promoted the most exciting body of research and discovery that medical science has ever known, but which now stands in the way of a progressive transition toward new insights and a new paradigm (Dixon, 1978).

The specific etiology paradigm: Its growth and decline

Many factors contributed to the growth of the specific etiology concept: the notion of contagion in the Bible with

its rules for ritual cleansing after contact with the "un-
clean"; the idea of quarantine with the forty-day separation
of those who had had contact with the bubonic plague; a
preoccupation with nosology, i.e., the systematization of
diseases according to their symptoms; the start of experimental medicine with the artificial creation of disease in
animals to determine what goes wrong in pathological
conditions. When Pasteur demonstrated unambiguously the
connection between specific microorganisms and their
specific effects and Koch established his rules for researching these effects, the truth of specific etiology was accepted beyond all reasonable doubt. Causative agents for at
least 22 infections were discovered before 1900 and the
dream of specific treatments for the indicted microbes grew.
When the theory that bacilli secreted toxins was vindicated, an antitoxin for diptheria was developed, and mathemati-
cally exact guidelines for standardizing bacterial toxins
and antitoxins were set forth by George Ehrlich who conceived of vaccines as magic bullets which could steer
straight to their targets: tuberculosis, cholera, typhoid. Ehrlich also introduced chemotherapy through his research
with chemical dyes to combat malaria and his success with
an arsenical No. 606, Salvarsan, against syphilis. The
arsenal of specific antidotes to specific diseases grew. The
notion of specific etiology was supported further when,
with the gradual discovery of vitamins, specific deficiency
diseases could be linked with specific vitamin or mineral
deficiencies as in rickets, tetany, night blindness, scurvy,
polyneuritis, pellagra, dermatitis and megaloblastic anemia. Specific etiology remained a fruitful paradigm for
research into genetic defects, hormone function, sickle cell
anemia and the localization of function in the brain.

Now, however, the fruitfulness of the notion of specif-
icity is withering as new data appear which cannot be
subsumed under its aegis and therefore demand a new
paradigm. Antibiotics, through reckless overuse, are no
longer specific for mutant, resistant strains of microorganisms and this resistance is contagious among other microorganisms. It also appears that other factors besides the

presence of microbes determine the outbreak of disease, i.e.,
the body's nutritional status, its ecological environment,
genetic constitution, age, stress, fatigue, mental attitude, the
virulence of the pathogen, the competence of the body's
immune reaction, the notion of biological individuality,
popularized by Roger Williams (1956) and now exquisitely
vindicated by the new knowledge of human leucocyte
antigens, HLA (Bylinsky, 1978). The now common knowledge that all microorganisms are not destructive, like those
in the gut which supply our B vitamins, weakens reliance
on a "magic bullet" and favors a policy of peaceful
coexistence with our microbe tenants.

What truly demolished the usefulness of specific
etiology is that it does not account for the major diseases of
our time, the degenerative diseases, heart disease, diabetes,
arthritis, rheumatism, allergies, cancer, mental illness.

Research into these diseases as governed by the
specific etiology paradigm merely leads up blind alleys and
turns health care into a science-fiction parts-repair workshop operated by a corps of medical traffic cops, each
watching his own corner—brain, eyes, nose-ear-throat,
heart, gut, ovary, rectum, bones, skin. No one bothers to
notice the whole person. The "mind" cop, a sort of
workshop receptionist, may exchange a few words as the
patients come and go to be checked up by the parts
policemen but he has no idea what parts are getting tested,
measured, patched up.

A life history of a not so mythical patient, M.P., would
run like this. M.P. feels pain in his big toe. Sees his
internist. Diagnosis: gout. Rx: medication, low purine diet.
M.P. experiences abdominal distress. Sees his gastroenter-
ologist. Diagnosis: colitis. Rx: sedatives, low residue diet.
M.P., aware of joint pains, tries an orthopedist who refers
him to a rheumatologist. Diagnosis: arthritis. By now he may
be grasping at any notion offering relief and may begin to
avoid what he considers acidic foods but succeeds only in
lowering his ascorbic acid intake. Tired and worried about
his health, he opts to see a cardiologist. Diagnosis: high
blood pressure and dysrhythmia. Rx: ease up, forego

strenuous exercise, plus low fat, low cholesterol and no eggs
and dairy products. Also he's given a heart stimulant and
a diuretic destined to deplete potassium and other mineral
stores. He feels weaker and more listless and discouraged.
Leaving the parts repair workshop, he stops to talk with the
receptionist mind cop. Diagnosis: masked depression,
psychosomatic somatizations (the official stamp of recognition that the mind can destroy but not that body metabolism influences thinking and feeling). Rx: more talk and a
musical chairs game of happy pills. After some time on
the psychotropic medication M.P. notes he has a tremor. He
sees the neurologist cop. Here he really gets tagged.
Diagnosis: Parkinsonism. Rx: L-dopa. Before the L-dopa can
lose its effectiveness M.P. saves face for his neuro cop by
having a stroke which now turns him into a baby-care-
package to be delivered to the terminal care nursing home
where his diet of sodawater and crackers will rapidly let
him be done in, mercifully, by cancer.

The red thread running through this science-fiction
nightmare is the nutritional ignorance of the parts patrol-
men. M.P.'s gout could be attributed less to a high purine
diet than to a lack of the enzymes and coenzymes, vitamins
and minerals, needed for its metabolism. Of these, pyridoxine which is known to participate in more than 50 metabolic pathways, is not only essential for protein metabolism
but appears to be of great relevance for all of M.P.'s
complaints. Lack of it is associated with kidney stones
(Sebrell, 1964; Gershoff, 1959). The same vitamin has also
been linked to cardiovascular disease by reason that a
deficiency leads to high levels of unconverted homocysteine
which directly aggravates placque formation (McCully,
1975). In this light it becomes apparent that M.P. was
iatrogenically programmed for the crescendo of his degenerative ailments.

This kingdom-for-a-horse parable is not meant to
imply any one-to-one relationship between a particular
essential vitamin (as is thought to exist in specific vitamin
deficiency diseases) and M.P.'s multifactorial diseases but
rather to decry the blinders that constrict the establish-

ment's vision to seeing only the symptoms as target rather
than the whole person-patient whose body needs a nutritional support system more than further attack and destruction. This is the cardinal sin committed in the name of the
specific etiology paradigm which has lost its utility.

Orthomolecular nutrition, the emergent paradigm

The paradigm that is replacing it is, of course, orthomolecular medicine because it fulfills the essential functions a
paradigm should by gathering, like butterflies in a net, all
the bits and pieces of widely diversified research and
human endeavor, and crystallizing them into a new image
of man. In addition, it gives direction, a more purposeful
direction, to further research.

Let me point out the signposts that show this is taking
place and perhaps dare to envision the direction that it
will go with just a pause to remind ourselves what this new
image of man is.

Man is more than a machine to be sliced up like a
sandwich into CAT scan slivers and then screwed together.
Man is, as Bertalanffy (1977), the general-systems theorist,
said, "an organized system" (Weiss, 1977). The wholeness
of the system is lost when attention to mere linear
causality blocks a systems-approach. A systems-approach
enhances our understanding of subcellular and cellular
relationships to their inner environment: the food and liquid
ingested for sustenance of the cellular structures, the air
breathed bringing life-sustaining oxygen or mood-altering
ionized particles (Soyka, 1978), or even potentially lethal
toxic molecules, the light that penetrating the eyes strikes
the pineal gland to affect the brain chemistry (Binkley,
1979; Wurtman, 1977b), the world beyond the senses (Smith,
1976) and rhythms that relate all of these together.

The cultural signposts are, like Gaul, tripartite: first, the
psychological phenomena, second, the biological-healing
phenomena, and third, the research phenomena. The notion

of expanded consciousness is the hallmark of the psychological phenomena. Contributing to it were Joseph Rhine's
research in ESP, the spread of Eastern psychology to the
West after the Communist destruction of Tibetan religion,
the mind-altering drugs of the drug culture, the populariza-
tion of alternative healing methods, and the establishment of
centers for their practice, the importation of Kirlian photog-
raphy from Russia, acupuncture from China, psychic healing
from the Philippines, books like *The Tao of Psychology*
(Bolen, 1979) and most significantly *The Tao of Physics*
(Capra, 1975) which uses the model of the most advanced
concepts in physics today to argue the identity not only
between man and his universe but with consciousness
itself. "The universal interwovenness always includes the
human observer and his or her consciousness, and this is
also true in atomic physics," says Capra. There is a move-
ment away from an objective monistic or dualistic view of
reality to one which encompasses the perceiver and also
allows for the same "reality" to be perceived as different
according to time and conditions in the same way as an
electron may be both a particle and a wave. The Indian
poet Tagore anticipated the modern mind-set more than half
a century ago: "One in the sense of Eastern mention, gold
and the bracelet, water and the wave."

The biological phenomena, like the psychological,
started in the early fifties with the birth of two opposing but
related forms of therapy for mental illness. Both acknowledged the illness as a brain disease that could be managed
by altering brain chemistry. The first of these in time was
orthomolecular psychiatry, then called megavitamin therapy
by its founders, Dr. Abram Hoffer and Dr. Humphry
Osmond. By one of those quirks of medical history, the
orthomolecular approach was soon overshadowed by the
advent of the second biological psychiatry method, psychotropic drugs. At last the mind was joined to its body, a
union that spurred research developments in brain chemistry and in neurotransmitter theory.

Orthomolecular research and prospects

Research today therefore reflects this conjunction of brain, body and the total environment. The medical geography studies, a new design in research, show the relationship between diet and health and behavioral factors in various discrete geographical areas of the world, between wheat and schizophrenia in Sweden (Dohan, 1966), between corn consumption and homicide in high-corn consuming areas (Mawson, 1978), between a low protein, high carbohydrate diet and aggressiveness among the Qolla (Bolton, 1978), between high selenium areas and freedom from cancer (Shamberger, 1976; Schrauzer, 1977), between soft water, depleted soils and heart disease (Punsar, 1978). Geographical pockets of longevity are also reported on.

A most stimulating field of research which is not only a pointed indicator of where we are but telegraphs the future is that which deals with the modulating effect of specific dietary factors on neurotransmitter levels and thus their influence on certain brain diseases. A simple illustration of this type of investigation is a study that shows that ascorbic acid enhances the release of acetylcholine and noradrenaline from synaptic vesicles (Kuo, 1979). But the leading researchers in this field are those working with Richard Wurtman in the Laboratory of Neuroendocrine Regulation, Department of Nutrition and Food Science at M.I.T. (Wurtman, 1977a). They have shown that oral choline can raise brain acetylcholine (Hirsch, 1978a, 1978b), a technique that has therapeutic value for patients with tardive dyskinesia (Growden, 1977a; Wurtman, 1978a), with Huntington's disease (Growden, 1977b; Wurtman, 1978b), or with premature memory loss (Davis, 1979; Sitaram, 1978). This last connection makes the loss of memory that accompanies tobacco withdrawal understandable since nicotine pathways are identical with acetylcholine pathways. By manipulating protein, fat and carbohydrate intake, these researchers have shown that brain serotonin levels can be shifted (Growden, 1977c; Fernstrom, 1971). Contrariwise, by altering brain serotonin levels by means of drugs, they were able to demonstrate a change in appetite for a preferential choice of protein or carbohydrate (Wurtman, 1979).

These limited references to current developments in the burgeoning research alliance between nutritional factors and the neurochemistry of mental functioning portends the future and brings psychiatry full circle away from an abortive interest in toximolecular pharmacological agents and back to the supportive measures of the orthomolecular approach pioneered by Hoffer and Osmond. This research direction, despite the complexity of the problems to be solved, holds great promise and infinite excitement. Consider some projects for the future: one, mapping out interrelationships of all nutritional building blocks, of enzymes and their cofactors with neurotransmitters and secondary transmitters known and as yet unknown to broaden the base for orthomolecular psychiatric practice; two, mapping out profile patterns for HLA antigens to identify persons genetically predisposed to particular degenerative or infectious diseases; three, fulfilling Linus Pauling's vision of developing blood and urine profiles for a hundred diseases to facilitate instant matching by computer with patient's samples. With such knowledge and screening devices medical practice will be primarily preventive and orthomolecular nutritional measures will be the means of providing for specific individual needs before the advent of disease.

What will be doctors' views of orthomolecular medicine then? Will there be any opponents left? Loren Mosher, one of the members of the APA Task Force once said that if every psychiatrist in the U.S.A. believed that megavitamin therapy helped schizophrenic patients, he would not believe it. His inflexibly rigid outlook reminds one of the character who visited an insane asylum and was bothered that the inmates looked so undistinguishable from the people outside. "How do you judge who is insane and who should be sent home?" he asked an attendant. "Oh, that's easy," replied the attendant. "Periodically we fill up that trough with water and give all the inmates a bucket and instruct them to empty the trough." "But how does that help you separate who stays and who goes home?" "Simple," retorted the attendant. "The first guy who turns off the faucet goes home." "Gosh," exclaimed the visitor, "I never thought of that."

A broadened vision is an asset also in recognizing orthomolecular medicine as the emergent medical paradigm.

Summary

The medical establishment's resistance to orthomolecular psychiatry follows predictable patterns common through-out medical history: ridiculing and denigrating the source of the new idea, refusing to examine the data, or doing so on a selective basis and making false representations about it, then defending one's avowed position by closing ranks in an "Old Boys' Club."

This was the same way in which the medical establish-ment dealt with Mendel, Schwann, Semmelweis, Pasteur, Florence Nightingale, Joseph Goldberger.

An idea that comes ahead of its time in medicine has to wait for the climate of opinion to change so that a new paradigm, or model of reality, is constructed. This paradigm gives direction to all forms of creativity and to scientific research.

Specific etiology is the paradigm that has held sway during a long period of productive research which achieved control over most of our contagious diseases, but the model no longer answers the needs of today's degenerative diseases, cancer, diabetes, heart disease, arthritis, rheuma-tism, allergies, mental illness. Actually, it misguides research.

The orthomolecular paradigm with its emphasis on optimum nutrition for the whole person takes a general systems approach that fits the developing climate of opinion which sees man as a unity within himself and within his ecology.

It is predictable that research stimulated by this emergent paradigm will concern itself with studies on nutrition, such as worldwide dietary patterns and their effects upon health and behavior, on HLA studies furthering our knowledge of genetically determined biological individuality, on Pauling's research into profiles of disease derived from body excretions, and particularly on studies relating specific nutritional factors to brain neurotransmitter effects. This approach will provide the basis for a true program for identifying disease and preventing it before it occurs, a real preventive medicine.

BIBLIOGRAPHY

Bertalanffy, L.V., 1977. The role of systems theory in present-day science, technology and philosophy. In: K.E. Schaefer, H. Hansel, R. Brady (Eds.): *Toward a Man-Centered Medical Science.* Mt. Kisko, New York: Futura Publ. Co.

Binkley, S. April, 1979. The time keeping enzyme in the pineal gland. *Scientific American* 66–71.

Bolen, J.S. 1979. *The Tao of Psychology: Synchronicity and the Self.* New York: Harper and Row.

Bolton, R. 1978. *Aggression in Qolla Society.* Champaign, Ill.: Garland Press.

Bylinsky, G. Sept. 25, 1978. A new power to predict—and prevent—disease. *Fortune* 108–115.

Capra, F. 1975. *The Tao of Physics.* Boulder, Co: Shambhala Publications.

Chalmers, T.C. Aug., 1977. Peer review of manuscripts. Letter, *New England Journal of Medicine* 297, 5, p. 285.

Cole, S., Rubin, L., and Cole, J. Oct., 1977. Peer review and the support of science. *Scientific American* 237, 4, 34–41.

Davis, K. and Yamamura, H.I. 1979. Cholinergic underactivity in human memory disorders. *Life Sciences* 23, 1729–1734.

Dixon, B. 1978. *Beyond the Magic Bullet.* New York: Harper and Row.

Dohan, F.C. 1966. Cereals and schizophrenia: data and hypothesis. *Acta Psychiatr. Scand.* 42, 125–152.

Fernstrom, J.D. and Wurtman, R.J. 1971. Brain serotonin content: increase following ingestion of carbohydrate diet. *Science* 174, 1023–1025.

Fishbein, M. 1967. Attitude and the prediction of behavior. In: Martin Fishbein (Ed.): *Readings in Attitude Theory and Measurement*. New York: John Wiley and Sons.

Gershoff, S.N. and Faragalla, F.F. 1959. *Journal of Biol. Chem.* 234, 2391–2393.

Good, R.A. 1979. Nutrition, immunity and cancer—a review. *Clinical Bulletin* 9, 1, 8–11.

Growden, J.H., Cohen, E.L. and Wurtman, R.J. 1979b. Effects of oral choline administration on serum and CSF choline levels in patients with Huntington's disease. *J. Neurochem.* 28, 229–231.

Growden, J.H., Cohen, E.L. and Wurtman, R.J. 1977c. Treatment of brain disease and dietary precursors of neurotransmitters. *Annals of Internal Medicine* 86, 337–339.

Growden, J.H., Hirsch, M.J., Wurtman, R.J. and Wiener, W. Sept. 8, 1977a. Oral choline administration to patients with tardive dyskinesia. *New England Journ. of Medicine* 297, 524.

Hawkins, D. and Pauling, L. 1973. *Orthomolecular Psychiatry*. San Francisco: W.H. Freeman and Co.

Hirsch, M.J., Growden, J.H. and Wurtman, R.J. August, 1978a. Relations between dietary choline or lecithin intake, serum choline levels, and various metabolic indices. *Metabolism* 27, 8.

Hirsch, M.J. and Wurtman, R.J. October 13, 1978b. Lecithin consumption increases acetylcholine concentration in rat brain and adrenal gland. *Science* 202 (4364), 223–225.

Hoffer, A. and Osmond, H. 1976. Megavitamin therapy, in reply to the American Psychiatric Association Task Force Report on megavitamin and orthomolecular therapy in psychiatry. Canadian Schizophrenia Foundation, 2229 Broad St., Regina, Saskatchewan, S4P1Y7.

Hospital Practice: Goldberger, Joseph. March, 1978. An unremitting struggle to conquer pellagra. *Hospital Practice* 13, 3, 136–164.

Kuhn, T.S. 1970. *The Structure of Scientific Revolutions*. 2nd Ed. Chicago: U. of Chicago Press.

Kuo, Che-Hui; Fumiaka, H.; Yoshida, H.; Yamatodani, A; and Wada, H. 1979. Effect of ascorbic acid on release of acetylcholine from synaptic vesicles prepared from different species of animals and release of noradrenaline from synaptic vesicles of rat brain. *Life Sciences* 24, 10, 911–916.

Mandell, Marshall. Personal communication.

Mawson, A.R. and Jacobs, K.W. 1978. Corn consumption, tryptophan, and cross-national homicide rates. *J. of Orthomolecular Psychiatry* 7, 4, 222–229.

McCully, K.S. and Wilson, R.B. 1975. Homocysteine theory of arteriosclerosis. *Atherosclerosis* 22, 215–227.

McGuire, W.J. 1967. Cognitive consistency and attitude change. In: Martin Fishbein (Ed.): *Readings in Attitude Theory and Measurement*. New York: John Wiley and Sons.

McGuire, W.J. 1973. Persuasion, resistance, and attitude change. In: Ithiel de Sola Pool, Wilbur Schramm (Eds.): *Handbook of Communication*. Chicago: Rand McNally.

Megavitamin and orthomolecular therapy in psychiatry: a report of the APA Task Force on vitamin therapy in psychiatry. Washington, American Psychiatric Association, 1973.

New York Times, October 3, 1979.

Pauling, L. April 19, 1968. Orthomolecular psychiatry. *Science* 160, 265–271.

Pauling, L. Personal communication, 1979.

Povolotsky, Y.L. and Krivokhatskaya, L.D. April, 1979. Effect of dibazol and ascorbic acid on antiviral activity of human interferon in cell culture. *Antibiotiki* 24, 4, 291–294.

Punsar, S. and Karvonen, M.J. 1978. Drinking water quality and sudden death: observations from west and east Finland. *Advances in Cardiology* 25, 25–26.

Rhine, B.J., 1967. A concept-formation approach to attitude acquisition. In: Martin Fishbein (Ed.): *Readings in Attitude Theory and Measurement*. New York: John Wiley and Sons.

Schrauzer, G. Paper presented at the Third International Symposium on Trace Element Metabolism in Man and Animals. Germany, Summer, 1977.

Sebrell, Jr., W.H. 1964. The importance of vitamin B6 in human nutrition. Paper presented at the International Symposium on Vitamin B6 in honor of Prof. Paul György. New York, July 23–24.

Shamberger, R., Tytko, S.A. and Willis, C.E. Sept.-Oct., 1976. Anti-oxidants and cancer. Pt. 6, selenium and age-adjusted human cancer mortality. *Archives of Environmental Health* 31, 231–235.

Siegel, B.V. 1974. Enhanced interferon response to murine leukemia virus by ascorbic acid. *Infect-Immunity* 10, 409.

Siegel, B.V. 1975. Enhancement of interferon production by poly (rl) poly (rC) in mouse cell cultures by ascorbic acid. *Nature* 254, p. 531, London.

Sitaram, N.; Weingartner, H.; Caine, E.D.; and Gillin, J.C. 1978. Choline: selective enhancement of serial learning and encoding of low imagery words in Man. *Life Sciences* 22, 17, 1555–1560.

Smith, H. 1976. *The Forgotten Truth: The Primordial Tradition.* New York: Harper and Row.

Stent, G.S. Dec., 1972. Prematurity and uniqueness in scientific discovery. *Scientific American,* 84–93.

Soyka, F. and Edmonds, A. 1978. *The Ion Effect.* New York: Bantam.

U.S. Government. Diet related to killer diseases, V: nutrition and mental health. Hearing before the Select Committee on Nutrition and Human Needs of the United States Senate, June 22, 1977. U.S. Government Printing Office, Washington, 1977.

Weiss, P.A. The system of nature and the nature of systems. Empirical holism and practical reductionism harmonized In: Schaefer, K.E., Hansel, H., Brady, R. (Eds.) *Toward a Man-Centered Medical Science.* Mt. Kisko, New York: Futura Publ. Co., 1977.

Williams, R.J. *Biochemical Individuality.* New York, John Wiley and Sons, 1956. Republished by U. of Texas Press, Austin and London, paperback, 1975.

Wurtman, R.J., Cohen, E.L. and Fernstrom, J.D. Control of brain neurotransmitter synthesis by precursor availability and food consumption In: Usdin, E. et al. (Eds.): *Neuroregulators and Psychiatric Disorders.* New York, Oxford U. Press, 103–121, 1977a.

Wurtman, R.J. and Moskowitz, M. June 9, 1977f. The pineal gland. *New England Journal of Medicine* 296, 23, 1329–1386.

Wurtman, R.J. 1978a. Relation between choline availability, acetycholine synthesis and cholinergic function. In: S. Garattini (Ed.): *Depressive Disorders*. Stuttgart, Schattauer.

Wurtman, R.J. and Growden, J.H. Dietary enhancement of CNS neurotransmitters. *Hospital Practice*, 71–77, March, 1978b.

Wurtman, J.J. and Wurtman, R.J. 1979. Drugs that enhance central serotoninergic transmission diminish carbohydrate consumption by Rats. *Life Sciences* 24, 10, 895–904.

SUGGESTED ADDITIONAL READING

Albanese, A. A.; Edelson, A. H.; Woodhull, M. L.; Lorzene, E. J., Jr.; Wein, E. H.; and Orto, L. A. 1973. Effect of calcium supplement on serum cholesterol, calcium, phosphorus, and bone density of "normal, healthy" elderly females. *Nutrition Reports International* 8:119–130.

Albrink, J. J., Davidson, P. C. and Newman, T. 1976. Lipid lowering effect of a very high carbohydrate high fiber diet. *Diabetes* 26 (Suppl. 1): 324.

Allaway, W. H.; Kubota, J.; Losee, F.; and Roth, M. 1968. Selenium, molybdenum, and vanadium in human blood. *Archives of Environmental Health* 16:342–348.

Allen, H. A. J. 1972. An investigation of water hardness, calcium and magnesium in relation to mortality in Ontario. Ph.D. thesis, University of Waterloo, Ontario, Canada.

Anderson, J. W. 1980. Dietary fiber in diabetes. In *Medical Aspects of Dietary Fiber*. Spiller, G. A. and Kay, R., eds. New York: Plenum Press.

—. 1977. Effect of carbohydrate restriction and high carbohydrate diets on men with chemical diabetes. *American Journal of Clinical Nutrition* 30:402–408.

—. 1977. High polysaccharide diet studies in patients with diabetes and vascular disease. *Cereal Foods World* 22:12–15.

Anderson, J. W. and Sieling, B. 1979. *HCF Diets: A User's Guide to High Carbohydrate High Fiber Diets.* Lexington, KY.: University of Kentucky Diabetes Research and Education Fund.

—. 1978. Long term effects of high carbohydrate, high fiber diets on glucose and lipid metabolism: a preliminary report on patients with diabetes. *Diabetes Care* 1:77082.

Anderson, J. W., Sieling, B. and Ferguson, S. 1979. Long term effects of high-fiber diets on mineral and fat soluble vitamin status in persons with diabetes. *Diabetes* 28:384.

Anderson, T. W. 1972. Serum electrolytes and skeletal mineralization in hard and soft-water areas. *Canadian Medical Association Journal* 107:34–37.

Anderson, T. W.; Neri, L. C.; Schreiber, G. B.; Talbot, F. D. F. and Zdrojewski, A. 1975. Ischemic heart disease, water hardness and myocardial magnesium. *Canadian Medical Association Journal* 113:199–203.

Arneson, G. A. 1964. Phenothiazine derivatives and glucose metabolism. *Journal of Neuropsychiatry* 5:191–195.

Basta, Lofty; Williams, Chad; Kioschos, J.; Michael, Spector; Arthur, A. 1976. Regression of atherosclerotic stenosing lesions of the renal arteries and spontaneous cure of systemic hypertension through control of hyperlipidemia. *The American Journal of Medicine* 61:420–423.

Bejerot, Nils. 1972. *Addiction—An Artificially Induced Drive.* Springfield: Charles C. Thomas.

Bell, Iris R. 1974. The kinin peptide hormone theory of adaptation and maladaptation in psychobiological illness. Ph.D. dissertation, Stanford University.

—. 1975. A kinin model of mediation for food and chemical sensitivities; Biobehavioral implications. *Annals of Allergy* 35:206:15.

Bennion, L. J. and Grundy, S. M. 1977. Effects of diabetes mellitus on cholesterol metabolism in man. *New England Journal of Medicine* 296:1365–1371.

Bersohn, I. and Oclofse, P. J. 1957. Correlation of serum magnesium and serum cholesterol levels in South African Bantu and European subjects. *Lancet* 1:1020–1021.

Bierenbaum, M. L., Fleischman, A. I. and Raichelson, R. I. 1972. Long term human studies on the lipid effects of oral calcium. *Lipids* 7:202–206.

Bierenbaum, M. L.; Fleischman, A. I.; Dunn, J. and Arnold, J. 1975. Possible toxic water factor in coronary heart disease. *Lancet* 1:1008–1010.

Bierenbaum, M. L.; Fleischman, A. I.; Dunn, J. P.; Hayton, T.; Pattison, D. C. and Watson, P. B. 1973. Serum parameters in hard and soft water communities. *American Journal of Public Health* 63:169–173.

Bland, Jeffrey. 1982. *The Accessory Nutrients* vols. 1 and 2. New Canaan, CT: Keats Publishing, Inc.

Bottazzo, G., et al. 1974. Islet-cell antibodies in diabetes mellitus with autoimmune polyendocrine deficiencies. *Lancet* 2:1279–1283.

Brown, J.; Bourke, G. J.; Gearty, G. F.; Finnegan, A.; Hill, M.; Heffernan-Fox, F. C.; Fitzgerald, D. E.; Kennedy, J.; Childers, R. W.; Jessop, W. J. E.; Trulson, M. F.; Latham, M. C.; Cornen, S.; McCann, M. B.: Clancy, R. E.; Gore, I.; Stoudt, H. W.; Hegsted, D. M. and Stare, F. J. 1970. Nutritional and epidemiologic factors related to heart disease. *World Review of Nutrition and Diet* 12:1–42.

Burkitt, D. P. 1978. Colonic-rectal cancer: fiber and other dietary factors. *American Journal of Clinical Nutrition* 31: S58–S64.

Burkitt, D. P. and Trowell, H. C. 1975. *Refined Carbohydrate Foods and Disease. Some Implications of Dietary Fibre.* New York: Academic Press.

Campbell, B. J.; Reinhold, J. G.; Cannell, J. J. and Nourmand, I. 1976. The effects of prolonged consumption of whole meal bread upon metabolism of calcium, magnesium, zinc and phosphorus of two young American adults. *Pahlavi Medical Journal* 7:1–7.

Canfield, W. K. and Doisy, R. J. eds. 1975. Evidence of an unrecognized metabolic defect in diabetic subjects. *Diabetes* 24 (2):406 (abstract).

—. 1976. Chromium and diabetes in the aged. In *The Biomedical Role of Trace Elements in Aging.* J. M. Hsu, R. L. Davis, and R.

W. Neithamer. St. Petersburg, Fla.: Eckerd College Gerontology Center, pp. 117–126.

Carlson, L. A.; Olsson, A. G.; Oro, L. and Rossner, S. 1971. Effects of oral calcium upon serum cholesterol and triglycerides in patients with hyperlipidemia. *Atherosclerosis* 14:391– 400.

Carr, C. J., Talbot, J. M. and Fisher, K. D. 1975. *A review of the significance of bovine milk xanthine oxidase in the etiology of atherosclerosis.* Bethesda Md.: Life Sciences Research Office, Federation of American Societies for Experimental Biology.

Carter, J. P.; Kattob, A.; Abd-El-Hadi, K.; Davis, J. T.; El Cholmy, A. and Pathwardhan, V. N. 1968. Chromium III in hypoglycemia and impaired glucose utilization in Kwashiorkor. *American Journal of Clinical Nutrition* 21:195–202.

Chase, H. P. and Glasgow, A. M. 1976. Juvenile diabetes mellitus and serum lipids and lipoprotein levels. *American Journal of Diseases of Children* 130:1113–1117.

Chipperfield, B. and Chipperfield, J. R. 1973. Heart-muscle magnesium, potassium, and zinc concentrations after sudden death from heart disease. *Lancet* 2:293–295.

Chipperfield, B.; Chipperfield, J. R.; Behr, G. and Burton, P. 1976. Magnesium and potassium content of normal heart muscle in areas of hard and soft water. *Lancet* 1:121–122.

Coca, A. F. 1942. *Familial Nonreagenic Food Allergy,* 1st ed. Springfield, IL: Charles C. Thomas.

Consolazio, C. F.; Matoush, L. O.; Nelson, R. A.; Harding, R. S. and Canham, J. E. 1962. Excretion of sodium, potassium, magnesium, and iron in human sweat and the relation of each to balance and requirements. *Journal of Nutrition* 19:407–415.

Cooper, Mildred and Cooper, Kenneth, H. 1977. *Aerobics for Women.* New York: Bantam Books.

Cotzias, G. C.; Horiuchi, K.; Fuenzalida, S. and Mena, I. 1968. Chronic manganese poisoning. *Neurology* 18:376–382.

Crawford, T. and Crawford, M. D. 1967. Prevalence and pathological changes of ischaemic heart-disease in a hard-water and in a soft-water area. *Lancet* 1:229–232.

Cummings, J. A. 1973. Dietary fibre. *Gut* 14:69–81.

Czerniejewski, C. P.; Shank, C. W.; Bechtel, W. G. and Bradley, W.

B. 1964. The minerals of wheat, flour, and bread. *Cereal Chemistry* 41:65–72.

Davidson, I. W. F. and Secrest, W. L. 1972. Determination of chromium in biological materials by atomic absorption spectrometry using a graphite furnace atomizer. *Analytical Chemistry* 44:1808–1813.

Davies, D. F.; Rees, B. W. G.; Johnson, A. P. and Elwood, P. C. 1974. Food antibodies and myocardial infarction. *Lancet* 1:1012–1014.

Dewar, J., Garcia-Webb, P., and Shenfield, G. M. 1979. Guar and diabetes. *Lancet* 1:612–614.

Doisy, R. J.; Streeten, D. H. P.; Freiberg, J. M. and Schneider, A. J. 1976. Chromium metabolism in man and biochemical effects. In *Trace Elements in Human Health and Disease*. A. Prasad, ed. New York: Academic Press, vol. 2, chap. 29.

Doisy, R. J.; Streeten, D. H. P.: Souma, M. L.; Kalafer, M. E.; Rekant, S. I. and Dalakos, T. G. 1971. Metabolism of chromium in human subjects. In *Newer Trace Elements in Nutrition*. W. Mertz and W. Cornatzer, eds. New York: Dekker, chap. 8.

Doisy, E. A., Jr. 1973. Micronutrient controls on biosynthesis of clotting proteins and cholesterol. In *Trace Substances in Environmental Health*. D. D. Hemphill, ed. Columbia: University of Missouri Press, vol. 6, pp. 193–199.

Dudley, E. F., Beldin, R. A. and Johnson, B. C. 1969. Climate, water hardness, and coronary heart disease. *Journal of Chronic Diseases* 22:25–48.

Ellenberg, M. 1977. Diabetes: Current status of an evolving disease. *New York State Journal of Medicine* 77:62–67.

Ellis, John M. November 12, 1972. Vitamin B6 in relation to diabetes mellitus. *Journal of the International Academy of Metabology* 11:1.

—. 1973. *Vitamin B6: The Doctor's Report*. New York: Harper and Row.

Elwood, P. C., Abernethy, M. and Morton, M. 1974. Mortality in adults and trace elements in water. *Lancet* 1470–1472.

Evans, G. W., Roginski, E. E. and Mertz, W. 1973. Interaction of the glucose tolerance factor (GTF) with insulin. *Biochemistry and Biophysics Research Community* 50:718–722.

Everson, G. J. and Shrader, R. E. 1968. Abnormal glucose tolerance in manganese-deficient guinea pigs. *Journal of Nutrition* 94:89–94.

Fleischman, Alan E.; Philpott, William H.; von Hilscheimer, G.; Moore, L.; Milner, P. N. and Klotz, S. D. 1974. Lipid chemistry and the psychiatric patient. *Journal of Orthomolecular Psychiatry* 4 (2):168–173.

Fox, M. R. S. 1970. The status of zinc in human nutrition. *World Review of Nutrition Diet* 12:208–226.

Freiberg, J. M.; Schneider, T. R.; Streeten, D. H. P. and Schneider, A. J. 1975. Effect of brewer's yeast on glucose tolerance. *Diabetes* 24 (2):433 (abstract).

Glinsmann, W. H. and Mertz. 1966. Effect of trivalent chromium on glucose tolerance. *Metabolism* 15:510–520.

Goodman, Joseph I. 1979. *Diabetes Without Fear*. New York: Avon.

Gresham, G. A. 1976. *Atherosclerosis* 23:379.

Griffith, G. and Hedge, B. 1959. Trace elements in cardiovascular disease. *Illinois Medical Journal* 115:12–13.

Griffiths, N. M. and Thompson, C. D. 1974. Selenium in whole blood of New Zealand residents. *New Zealand Medical Journal* 80:199–205.

Gurson, C. T. and Saner, G. 1971. Effect of chromium on glucose utilization in marasmic protein-calorie malnutrition. *American Journal of Clinical Nutrition* 24:1313.

Guthrie, B. E. 1975. Chromium, manganese, copper, zinc, and cadmium content of New Zealand foods. *New Zealand Medical Journal* 82:418–424.

Halsted, J. A., Smith, J. C., Jr. and Irwin, M. I. 1975. A conspectus of research on zinc requirements of man. *Journal of Nutrition* 104:347–378.

Hambidge, J. M. 1971. Chromium nutrition in the mother and the growing child. In *Newer Trace Elements in Nutrition*. W. Mertz and W. E. Cornatzer, eds. New York: Dekker, chap. 9.

Hambidge, K. M.; Hambidge, C.; Jacobs, M. and Baum, J. D. 1972. Low levels of zinc in hair, anorexia, poor growth, and hypogeusia in children. *Pediatric Research* 6:868–874.

Hankin, J. H., Margen, S. and Goldsmith, N. F. 1970. Contribution of hard water to calcium and magnesium intakes of adults. *Journal of the American Dietetic Association* 56:212–224.

Harman, D. 1965. Atherosclerosis: Possible role of drinking water copper. *Clinical Research* 13:91.

Hedge, B., Griffith, G. C. and Butt, E. M. 1961. Tissue and serum manganese levels in evaluation of heart muscle damage. A comparison with SGOT. *Proceedings of the American Societies of Experimental Biology and Medicine* 107:734–737.

Higginbottom, M. C., Sweetman, L. and Nyham, W. L. 1978. A syndrome of methylmalonic aciduria, homocystinuria, megaboblastic anemia and neurological abnormalities in a vitamin B12 deficient breast-fed infant of a strict vegetarian. *New England Journal of Medicine* 299:317–323.

Holloway, W. D., Tasman-Jones, C. and Lee, S. P. 1978. Digestion of certain fractions of dietary fiber in humans. *American Journal of Clinical Nutrition* 31:927–930.

Hopkins, L. L., Jr., Ransome-Kuti, O. and Majaf, A. S. 1968. Improvement of impaired carbohydrate metabolism by chromium III in malnourished infants. *American Journal of Clinical Nutrition* 21:203–211.

Hsia, S. L.; Fishman, L. M.; Briese, F. W.; Christakes, G.; Burr, J. and Bricker, L. A. 1978. Decreased serum cholesterol binding reserve in diabetes mellitus. *Diabetes Care* 89–93.

Ismail-Beigi, F., Faraji, B. and Reinhold, J. G. 1977. Binding of zinc and iron to wheat bread, wheat bran, and their components. *American Journal of Clinical Nutrition* 30:1721–1725.

Jenkins, D. J. A.; Leeds, A. R.; Gassull, M. A.; Cochet, B. and Alberti, K. G. M. M. 1977. Decrease in postprandial insulin and glucose concentrations by guar and pectin. *Annals of Internal Medicine* 86:20–23.

Jenkins, D. J. A.; Wolever, T. M. S.; Hockaday, T. D. R.; Leeds, A. R.; Howarth, R.; Bacon, S.; Apling, E. C.; and Dilawari, J. 1977. Treatment of diabetes with guar gum. *Lancet* 2:779–780.

Jenkins, D. J. A.; Leeds, A. R.; Gassull, M. A.; Wolever, T. M. S.; Goff, D. V.; Alberti, K. G. M. M. and Hockaday, T. D. R. 1976. Unabsorbable carbohydrates and diabetes: decreased post-prandial hyperglycemia. *Lancet* 2:172–174.

Johnson, Joseph E. 1977. The role of infection in allergic disease. *Annual Review of Allergy.* 1975–1976. Claude Albee Frazier, M.D., ed. Flushing, New York: Medical Examination Publishing Company, pp. 434–442.

Kanabrocki, E. L.; Case, L. F.; Graham, L.; Fields, T.; Miller, E. B.; Oester, Y. T.; and Kaplan, E. 1967. Non-dialyzable manganese and copper levels in serum of patients with various diseases. *Journal of Nuclear Medicine* 8:166–172.

Karppanen, H. and Neuvonen, P. J. 1973. Ischemic heart-disease and soil magnesium in Finland. *Lancet* 2:1390.

Kay, R. M. and Strasberg, S. M. 1978. Origin, chemistry, physiological effects and clinical importance of dietary fibre. *Clinical Investigations* 1:9–24.

Keys, A. 1975. Coronary heart disease—the global picture. *Atherosclerosis* 22:149–192.

Kiehm, Tae G., Anderson, James W. and Ward, Kyleen. 1976. Beneficial effects of a high carbohydrate, high fiber diet on hyperglycemic diabetic men. *American Journal of Clinical Nutrition* 29:895–899.

Klevay, L. M. 1975. Coronary heart disease: The zinc/copper hypothesis. *American Journal of Clinical Nutrition* 28:764–774.

Klevay, L. M. 1973. Hypercholesterolemia in rats produced by an increase in the ratio of zinc to copper ingested. *American Journal of Clinical Nutrition* 26:1060–1068.

Kobayashi, J. 1972. Air and water pollution by cadmium, lead and zinc attributed to the largest zinc refinery in Japan. In *Tract Substances in Environmental Health,* D. D. Hemphill, ed. Columbia: University of Missouri, vol. 5, pp. 117–128.

Kostrubala, Thaddeus. 1976. *The Joy of Running.* Philadelphia and New York: Lippincott.

Leonard, Jon N., Jofer, J. S., Pritikin, N. 1977. *Live Longer Now.* New York: Grosset and Dunlap.

Levine, R. A., Streeten, D. H. P. and Doisy, R. J. 1968. Effects of oral chromium supplementation on the glucose tolerance of elderly human subjects. *Metabolism* 17:114–125.

Libby, A. F. and Stone, Irwin. 1977. The hypoascorbemia-kwashiorkor approach to drug addiction therapy: a pilot study. *Journal of Orthomolecular Psychiatry* 6 (4):300–308.

Lindemann, R. D. and Assenzo, J. R. 1964. Correlations between water hardness and cardiovascular deaths in Oklahoma counties. *American Journal of Public Health* 54:1071–1077.

Linder, A.; Charra, B.; Sherrard, D. J. and Scribner, B. H. 1974. Accelerated atherosclerosis in prolonged maintenance hemodialysis. *New England Journal of Medicine* 290:697–701.

Livingston, Afton Monk; Livingston, Virginia Wuerthele-Caspe; Alexander Jackson, Eleanor and Wolter, Gerhard H. 1980. Toxic fractions obtained from tumor isolated and related clinical implications. *Annals of the New York Academy of Sciences* 174:2.

Maccuish, A., et al. December 1976. Antibodies to pancreatic islet cells in insulin-dependent diabetics with co-existent autoimmune disease. *Lancet* 2:1529–1531 (no. 7896).

Matrone, G. 1974. Chemical parameters in trace element antagonisms. In *Trace Element Metabolism in Animals.* W. G. Hoekstra, J. W. Suttie, H. E. Ganther and W. Mertz, eds. Baltimore: University Park Press, vol. 2, pp. 91–103.

Maxia, V.; Meloni, S.; Rollier, M. A.; Brandone, A.; Parwardhan, V.; Waslien, C. I. and El Shami, S. 1972. Selenium and chromium assay in Egyptian foods and in blood of Egyptian children by activation analysis. In *Nuclear Activation Techniques in the Life Sciences. IAEA 157/67.* Vienna: International Atomic Energy Agency.

McKenzie, M. M. and Kay, D. L. 1973. Urinary excretion of cadmium, zinc and copper in normotensive and hypertensive women. *New Zealand Medical Journal* 80:68–70.

McNamara, J. J.; Molot, M. A.; Stremple, J. F. and Cutting, R. F. 1971. Coronary artery disease in combat casualties in Vietnam. *JAMA* 216:1185–1187.

Mertz, W. 1967. Biological role of chromium. *Federation Proceedings* 26:186–193.

Mertz, W., Roginski, E. E. and Schwarz, K. 1961. Effect of trivalent chromium complexes on glucose uptake by epididymal fat tissue of rats. *Journal of Biological Chemistry* 226:318–322.

Mervyn, L. 1981. *Minerals and Your Health.* New Canaan, CT: Keats Publishing, Inc.

Miranda, P. M. and Horwitz, D. I. High fiber diets in the treatment of diabetes mellitus. *Annals of Internal Medicine* 88:482–486.

Moore, L. A., Hallman, E. T. and Sholl, L. B. 1938. Cardiovascular and other lesions in calves fed diets low in magnesium. *Archives of Pathology* 1:820–838.

Morgan, J. M. 1972a. Hepatic chromium content in diabetic subjects. *Metabolism* 21:313–316.

Moynahan, E. J. 1974. Acrodermatitis enteropathica: a lethal inherited human zinc-deficiency disorder. *Lancet* 2:399–400.

Muth, O. H.; Weswig, P. H.; Whanger, P. D. and Oldfield, J. E. 1971. Effect of feeding selenium-deficient ration to the subhuman primate Saimiri sciureus. *American Journal of Veterinary Research* 32:1603–1605.

Neldner, K. H. and Hambidge, K. M. 1975. Zinc therapy of acrodermatitis enteropathica. *New England Journal of Medicine* 292:879–881.

Noller, H. G. 1962. Results of examinations of stomach functions with the endo-radio capsule—the heidelberg capsule—a new appliance for assisting stomach diagnosis. *Fortschritte der Medizin* 80:351.

Oberleas, D., Harland, B. F. and Connor, D. H. 1976. Some metabolic hazards of elevated dietary fiber intake. *Federal Proceedings* 35 (3):343 (abstract).

O'Dell, B. L., Morris, E. R. and Regan, W. O. 1960. Magnesium requirement of guinea pigs and rats. Effects of calcium and phosphorus and symptoms of magnesium deficiency. *Journal of Nutrition* 70:103–111.

Palumbo, P. J., Briones, E. R. and Nelson, R. A. 1978. High fiber diet in hyperlipemia. *JAMA* 240:223–227.

Passwater, R. and Cranton, E. M. 1982. *Trace Elements, Hair Analysis and Nutrition.* New Canaan, CT: Keats Publishing, Inc.

Pfeiffer, C. C. 1975. *Mental and Elemental Nutrients.* New Canaan, CT: Keats Publishing, Inc.

Philpott, William H. 1974. Method of deliberate food testing for emotional reactions. *Journal of Orthomolecular Psychiatry* 111 (3):186–195.

—. 1974. Ecologic, orthomolecular and behavioral contributions to psychiatry. *Journal of Orthomolecular Psychiatry* 111(4):356–370.

—. 1976 Methods of relief of acute and chronic symptoms of deficiency-allergy-addiction maladaptive reactions to foods and chemicals. In *Clinical Ecology*. Lawrence Dickey, ed. Springfield, IL: Charles C. Thomas, pp. 496–509.

Potts, John and Lang, Melvin S. 1977. Avoidance provocative food testing in assessing diabetes responsiveness. *Diabetes* 26.

Pritikin, Nathan. 1976. High carbohydrate diets: maligned and misunderstood. *Journal of Applied Nutrition* 28:56–68.

Randolph, T. G. 1976. Adaptation to specific environmental exposures enhanced by individual susceptibility. *Clinical Ecology*, Lawrence Dickey, ed. Springfield, IL: Charles C. Thomas, pp. 46–66.

—. 1976. Historical development of clinical ecology. *Clinical Ecology*, pp. 9–17.

—. June 1961. Ecologic mental illness—levels of central nervous system reactions. *Proceedings of the Third World Congress of Psychiatry*. Montreal, Canada: University of Toronto Press vol. 1, pp. 379–384.

—. March/April 1964. The Ecologic Unit, Part 1 and Part II. *Hospital Management*.

—. 1974. *The History of Ecologic Mental Illness*. In annual review of *Allergy 1973*. Claude Albee Frazier, ed. Flushing, New York: Medical Examination Publishing, pp. 425–441.

Rowe, A. M. 1931. *Food Allergies: Its Manifestations, Diagnosis and Treatment*. Philadelphia: Lea and Febiger.

—. 1944. Clinical allergy in the nervous system. *Journal of Nervous and Mental Disease* 99:834.

Sandstead, H. H. 1973. Zinc nutrition in the United States. *American Journal of Clinical Nutrition* 26:1251–1260.

Saner, G. 1975. Urinary chromium excretion in the newborn and its relation to intravenous glucose loading. *Nutrition Reports International* 11:387–392.

Saudek, C. D. and Brach, E. L. 1978. Cholesterol metabolism in diabetes. The effect of diabetic control on sterol balance. *Diabetes* 27:1059–1064.

Schroeder, H. A. 1966. Municipal drinking water and cardiovascular death rates. *Journal of the American Medical Association* 195:81–85.

—. 1968. The role of chromium in mammalian nutrition. *American Journal of Clinical Nutrition* 21:230–244.

Schroeder, H. A., Balassa, J. J. and Tipton, I. H. 1962. Abnormal trace metals in man: Chromium. *Journal of Chronic Diseases* 15:941–964.

—. 1963. Abnormal trace metals in man: Vanadium. *Journal of Chronic Diseases* 16:1047–1071.

Schroeder, H. A. and Buckman, J. 1967. Cadmium hypertension—its reversal in rats by a zinc chelate. *Archives of Environmental Health* 14:693–697.

Schroeder, H. A. and Kraemer, L. A. 1974. Cardiovascular mortality, municipal water and corrosion. *Archives of Environmental Health* 28:303–311.

Schroeder, H. A., Nason, A. P. and Tipton, I. H. 1970. Chromium deficiency as a factor in atherosclerosis. *Journal of Chronic Diseases* 23:123–142.

Schroeder, H. A.; Nason, A. P.; Tipton, I. H. and Balassa, J. J. 1967. Essential trace metals in man: Zinc. Relation to environmental cadmium. *Journal of Chronic Diseases* 20:179–210.

Schroeder, H. A. and Nason, A. P. 1976. Interactions of trace metals in mouse and rat tissues: Zinc, chromium, copper and manganese with 13 other elements. *Journal of Nutrition* 106:198–203.

Schwartz, K. and Mertz, W. 1959. Chromium III and the glucose tolerance factor. *Archives of Biochemistry and Biophysics* 85:292–295.

Seelig, M. S. and Heggtveit, H. A. 1974. Magnesium interrelationship in ischemic heart disease. A review. *American Journal of Clinical Nutrition* 27:59–79.

Seelig, M. S. 1964. The requirement of magnesium by the normal adult. *American Journal of Clinical Nutrition* 14:342–390.

Seltzer, H. S. 1979. Diagnosis of diabetes. In *Diabetes Mellitus: Theory and Practice*. M. Ellenberg and H. Rifkin, eds. New York: McGraw-Hill, pp. 436–507.

—. 1971. Oral glucose tolerance tests. In *Diabetes Mellitus: Diagnosis and Treatment*. S. S. Fajans and K. E. Sussman, eds. New York: American Diabetes Association, vol. III, pp. 101–106.

Selye, Hans. 1956. *The Stress of Life*. New York: McGraw-Hill.

Shamberger, R. J. and Willis, C. E. 1976. Epidemiological studies on selenium and heart disease. *Federation Proceedings* 35 (3):578 (abstract).

Sharrett, A. R. and Feinleib, M. 1975. Water constituents in relation to cardiovascular disease. *Preventive Medicine* 4:20–36.

Southgate, D. A. T.; Branch, W. J.; Hill, M. J.; Draser, B. S.; Walters, R. L.; Davies, P. S. and Baird, I. M. 1976. Metabolic responses in dietary supplements of bran. *Metabolism* 25: 1129–1135.

Spiller, G. A. and Amen, R. J. 1976. *Fiber in Human Nutrition.* New York: Plenum Press.

Stiles, L. W.; Rivers, J. M.; Hackler, L. R. and Van Campen, D. 1976. Altered mineral absorption in the rat due to dietary fiber. *Federation Proceedings* 35 (3):744 (abstract).

Subak-Sharpe, Genell. 1978. Know diabetes and know medicine. *Drug Therapy* 8:22–23.

Thonnard, Normann E. 1968. Phenothiazines and diabetes in hospitalized women. *American Journal of Psychiatry* 124: 982–987.

Tintera, John W. 1966. Stabilizing homeostasis in the recovered alcoholic through endocrine therapy: Evaluations of the hyperglycemic factor. *Journal of the American Geriatric Society* 14:126–148.

Trowell, H. C. 1976. Definition of dietary fiber and hypothesis that it is a protective factor in certain diseases. *American Journal of Clinical Nutrition* 29:417–427.

—. 1978. Diabetes mellitus and dietary fiber of starchy foods. *American Journal of Clinical Nutrition* 31:553–557.

Trowell, H. and Burkitt, D. 1977. Dietary fiber and cardiovascular disease. *Artery* 3:107–119.

Tuman, R. W. 1975. Biological effects of glucose tolerance factor (GTF) and inorganic chromium (III) in normal and genetically diabetic mice. Ph.D. thesis, State University of New York, Upstate Medical Center, Syracuse, New York.

Van Campen, D. R. 1966. Effects of zinc, cadmium, silver and mercury on the absorption and distribution of copper 64 in rats. *Journal of Nutrition* 88:125–130.

Van Campen, D. and Gross, E. 1968. Influence of ascorbic acid on the absorption of copper by rats. *Journal of Nutrition* 95:617–622.

Van Soest, P. J. and Robertson, J. B. 1977. What is fiber and fiber in food? *Nutrition Review* 35:12–16.

Venchikov, A. I. 1974. Zones of display of biological and pharmacotoxicological action of trace elements. In *Trace Element Metabolism in Animals*. W. G. Hoekstra; J. W. Suttie; H. E. Garther and W. Mertz, eds. Baltimore: University Park Press, pp. 295–310.

Voors, A. W. 1969. Does lithium depletion cause atherosclerotic heart disease? *Lancet* 2:1337–1339.

—. 1970. Lithium in the drinking water and atherosclerotic heart death: Epidemiologic argument for protective effect. *American Journal of Epidemiology* 92:164–171.

Waitzkin, L. 1966. A survey of unknown diabetics in a mental hospital. *Diabetes* 15:97–104.

Wapnick, S.; Wicks, A. C. B.; Kanengoni, E. and Jones, J. J. 1972. Can diet be responsible for the initial lesion in diabetes? *Lancet* 2:300–301.

West, K. M. and Kalbfleisch, J. M. 1971. Influence of nutritional factor on prevalence of diabetes. *Diabetes* 20:99–108.

Winegrad, Albert I. and Greene, Douglas A. 1976. Diabetic polyneuropathy: The importance of insulin deficiency, hyperglycemia and alterations in myoinosital metabolism in its pathogenesis. *New England Journal of Medicine* 295:1416–1420.

Wolf, Max and Ransberger, Karl. 1972. *Enzyme Therapy*. Los Angeles: Regent House.

Wolf, W., Mertz, W. and Masironi, R. 1974. Determination of chromium in refined and unrefined sugars by oxygen plasma ashing flameless atomic absorption. *Journal of Agricultural and Food Chemistry* 22:1037–1042.

INDEX

INDEX

Acidophilus bacteria
supplementation, for
bowels, 111
Addiction, 38–39, 40, 42
acidic state of, 31
adaptive, 38–39
definition of, 38
degenerative diseases
evoked by, 29
to self-produced narcotics,
32
withdrawal phase symptoms
of, 30, 38, 40
Adrenal cortex, 52
Adrenal medulla, 52
Africans
dietary fat of, and freedom
from atherosclerosis and
heart attacks, 131
dietary fiber among, and
low incidence of diabetes,
105–106

Aging, cellular, 172
Air pollution, maladaptive
reactions to, 74–75
Alcohol
avoidance of, in purposeful
violation of diversified
rotation diet, 99
and pancreatic insufficiency,
23
Alfalfa tablets, 112
Aloe vera, liquid, 69
Alpha cells, 56
Alpha-endorphins, 30–31
Alpha-ketoglutaric acid, low,
239–240
Altenburger, E., 144
Alvarez, W. C., 24
Ames, S. R., 173
Amino acid deficiency, 59–60,
65, 66, 77
Amino acid supplementation,
67–68, 70, 78, 99, 239–240